T0234276

Modeling Reality with Mathematics

Alfio Quarteroni

Modeling Reality
with
Mathematics

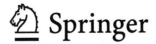 Springer

Alfio Quarteroni
École Polytechnique Fédérale de Lausanne (EPFL)
Lausanne, Switzerland

Politecnico di Milano
Milan, Italy

Translated by
Simon G. Chiossi
Departamento de Matemática Aplicada
Universidade Federal Fluminense
Niterói, Rio de Janeiro, Brazil

Translation from the Italian language edition: "Le equazioni del cuore, della pioggia e delle vele. Modelli matematici per simulare la realtà" by Alfio Quarteroni, © Zanichelli 2020. Published by Zanichelli. All Rights Reserved.

ISBN 978-3-030-96164-0   ISBN 978-3-030-96162-6   (eBook)
https://doi.org/10.1007/978-3-030-96162-6

This Springer imprint is published by the registered company Springer Nature Switzerland AG.
The registered company address is: Gewerbestrasse 11, 6330 Cham, Switzerland

to Lara, Luca, and Bianca Sofia,
my little models

Preface

Following the dramatic spread of the COVID-19 pandemic at the start of 2020, mathematics has never been so much at the centre of everybody's attention.

Expressions like *exponential, logistic function, extrema* and *inflection*, which until that moment we thought were confined to classrooms and university halls, all of a sudden have entered the political debate. This was all the more true in the initial stages of the epidemic, which were characterised by a major uncertainty regarding the contagion's evolution.

Yet even a casual observer must have noticed that mathematics is present in an increasingly pervasive way in our daily lives. There is chatter in the media about intangible algorithms for finding a soulmate, concocting the perfect diet or taking any decision whatsoever. The news report of billions of euros going up in flames on stock exchanges around the world due to an algorithm that went amok. They boast how *big data* (which everybody talks about, although very few truly know about) is essential for economic and technological advancement.

In this book, as you may have gathered from the title, I intend to present a version of mathematics that is less hostile and obscure. Or rather, I will present an area, called mathematical modelling, that over the last few decades has taken the front row. Whether we are aware of it or not (as is more often the case), we all regularly benefit from mathematical models and algorithms, and without them our lives would be very different. Here are some examples. Without mathematical models we would not know what the weather will look like tomorrow. We would not be able to share photos and videos on our phones, nor browse the web as fast as we do. We could not blindly rely on sat-navs to find our way through cities we have never been to before. Our cars would not be so silent, comfortable and efficient. We could not use CAT scans to take a look inside our bodies, nor would our favourite football team have a legion of *match analysts* studying strategies to boost competitiveness using the omnipresent *big data*. The list of similar stunning achievements could go on and on.

Mathematics is—even if you do not know, it is easy to guess so—an abstract science. And that is precisely one of its secret weapons. Abstraction allows us to study problems in their full generality, and helps us understand their key and innermost features. Abstraction tickles our imagination and imagination nurtures creativity, which in turn allows us to discover the best path towards solving our problems. We rely on abstraction to formulate far-fetching conjectures, which sometimes are so intricate that they withstand our attempts to solve (or disprove) them for centuries. Fermat's last theorem, for instance, was stated in 1637 and only proved by the British mathematician Andrew Wiles in 1994. The Riemann hypothesis was first published in 1859 and is still unsolved.

Mathematical models are characterised by being concrete, because they need to be both useful and of broad interest. As strange as it may sound, they are born and they flourish precisely because of abstraction. To better understand this crucial fact and reveal it in all its might, in the next pages we shall attempt to clarify what a mathematical model truly is, and present some examples.

Before that, though, we should recall the pivotal role of two core players in mathematics, which all of us have met in school, namely numbers and equations. *Numbers* allow us to quantify distances, weights, time intervals and so on. *Equations* describe in a general way the relationships that govern natural processes (the movement of a glacier, the flooding caused by a river's surge, the propagation of seismic waves but also solar combustion and even how a forest grows). Equations allow us to compute the trajectories of satellites and the courses of Formula 1 racing cars; they manage industrial processes and regulate the negotiation of complex financial instruments. Because of equations we are able to produce wonderful animated films (whose characters and events, albeit amazingly realistic, are solutions to mathematical equations), we can study the best tactic for a volleyball team and we can even simulate how vital organs like the heart or the brain work. All of this is possible because equations translate into symbols and mathematical relations physical laws, biological processes and social behaviours. In this way, they allow us to construct a virtual world (the model) starting from the real world. By solving equations we can make predictions (think of weather forecasts), simulate the progression of an illness or calculate how a volcanic eruption will disperse its ashes in the atmosphere. Summing up, a mathematical model's equations are telescopes pointed into the future.

Mathematics is the oldest among the sciences (the earliest written documents were found in ancient Egypt and Mesopotamia roughly 2000 BCE), and we can bet on it being the one that will survive them all. Mathematics is the only field capable of developing autonomously, since all other sciences require the language and the tools of mathematics to express themselves. We had better acknowledge its role then. If you are willing to accompany me on this journey, I intend to help you look at mathematics through a different lens. Hopefully, I will awaken (once more?) the interest of those of you who "In school I did understand maths, but there was a teacher who made me hate it." (In everyone's life there is always a teacher who made us love or hate a subject.)

So let the adventure begin: enjoy!

Milan, Italy, 2022   Alfio Quarteroni

Acknowledgements

I wish to thank my colleagues:

- Luca Bonaventura for the chapter WEATHER FORE-CAST MODELS
- Luca Dede' and Christian Vergara for the chapter A MATHEMATICAL HEART
- Nicola Parolini for the chapter MATHEMATICS IN THE WIND
- Gilles Fourestey, Nicola Parolini, Christophe Prud-homme and Gianluigi Rozza for the chapter FLYING ON SUN POWER
- Luca Paglieri for the chapter THE TASTE FOR MATHEMATICS.

A special thank to Francesca Bonadei from Springer Milan: her help and support are greatly appreciated.

Contents

List of Figures

1

The Model, aka the Magic Box

Abstract A mathematical model works like a box. The researcher puts in the data, the observations and the measurements, and the box returns the solutions to the model, that is, the expected values of the physical quantities describing the phenomenon.

In the past few days it has rained a lot and the river is full of water. How do we predict whether it will burst and flood the town centre?

There is no time to waste and we must act swiftly. We cannot study the river's behaviour for hours and try and guess what will happen. Neither can we base ourselves on similar past events, because floods are not a phenomenon that repeats itself cyclically and regularly. There are many random circumstances making every occurrence different from the previous ones.

We must know in advance the water's level at various points along the river to understand if and when it will

© The Author(s), under exclusive license to Springer Nature Switzerland AG 2022
A. Quarteroni, *Modeling Reality with Mathematics*,
https://doi.org/10.1007/978-3-030-96162-6_1

1

overflow. We need, in other terms, a sensible and fast prediction. Can we rely on mathematics for this? And how, exactly?

Let us think of the case at hand, the river's tipping point. We will need to know the following set of data:

- the shape of the river bed;
- the flow rate outside the city;
- how rough the surface of bed and banks is.

Now, before we start formulating the model's equations, we should determine which variables (the problem's solutions, or unknowns) describe in the most comprehensive way the process we want to examine. In our case we would like the model to provide the following (unknown) quantities:

- the speed of the flood wave at every point along the river course and at every instant in the successive hours;
- the water pressure at each point and at each instant of time (in particular, the pressure on the river banks);
- the shape of the wave's surface, which in turn will give us the water level reached at each point of the basin, at each time. (From that we will deduce if and when the river will burst.)

These solutions will be expressible in terms of mathematical functions, which are laws associating to each point in space and to each instant the numerical value of the following quantities:

- the speed (measured in metres per second);
- the pressure (in newtons);
- the elevation of the water crest (in metres).

(Note that if we had considered a water pipe instead of a river, like those downstream mountain dams, the unknowns would be the speed and the pressure. It would not make sense to consider the elevation, since one could assume that in a full pipe the water adheres to the inner walls.)

Now that we have established the data and the unknown variables, the model describing the physical phenomenon (the water flow, in our case) should allow us to pass from the data to the solutions. It does so thanks to equations, which are equalities between algebraic expressions that mathematically encode the relevant physical laws (fluid dynamics, in particular of water) and link the unknown quantities (the *solutions*) to the known ones (the *data*).

Often, physical laws are based on universal principles, such as conservation laws. Let us consider for instance the conservation of mass. In our case it translates into the conservation of the total quantity of water contained in a certain portion of the river basin. Consider the water mass contained in a 100 m stretch at 1 pm. It will equal the mass present at 12 pm, plus the water that flowed in upstream, minus the water that flowed out either downstream or from the banks in case of an outburst, during this hour. Or let us consider the conservation of force: in order to respect it, we will have to impose that the product of the water mass times its acceleration equals the sum of all forces acting on the water.

And that is not the end: other laws will impose further relationships/equations.

The real challenge is to express these laws on an infinitesimal volume of fluid, which in a limiting process becomes a point. Mathematically speaking, in fact, these laws describe the rate of change of the quantities involved in space and time. More precisely, they describe infinitesimal variations, meaning variations that are as small as we want.

A variation is just a difference: when we fall ill and our body temperature rises from 37 to 38 °C we say there has been a variation of one degree. If our firm's revenue last year jumped from 90 k to 100 k Euros, we say there was a variation of 10,000 Euros, and so forth. If we introduce a dynamical factor, and pass from an absolute variation to a variation measured against time, we obtain a rate of change. When the reference time intervals become smaller and smaller, we obtain the infinitesimal rate of change.

The most familiar example is probably measuring speed on a motorway. Suppose it takes us 5 minutes to drive between two speeding cameras placed 10 km apart. The system will record an *average speed* of 120 km/h (5 minutes correspond to 1/12 of an hour). To measure the *instantaneous speed* at a given point, instead, which is what we read on the dashboard, ideally we should bring the cameras closer, until their positions coincide. This is the practical rendition of a mathematical procedure called *limit*: the instantaneous speed is the limit value of the speeds measured over increasingly smaller travel times. Speed is an example of what in mathematics we call a *derivative*, a function that expresses the rate of change of the initial quantity. (If these notions are still a bit obscure, be patient; in a short while we will clarify them with concrete examples.)

Since change rates are expressed by derivatives, the model's equation will contain relationships between the solutions and their derivatives. These types of equations are called *differential equations*.

1.1   Initial Data

Suppose we are addressing, as in this case, a *dynamical model*, or *evolution model*, which describes a changing situation. In order to make predictions on future behaviours, it is necessary to include in the data the system's *initial state*. In our example this entails knowing the water's speed and depth at any point of the river bed at time zero. *Time zero* refers to the instant at which the simulation of the process is supposed to begin. For example, if we observe the water flow from today at 12 pm (time zero) until tomorrow at 12 pm (final time), in principle we would also need the full knowledge of the water's speed and depth at today's 12 pm. This would be if we lived in an idealised world. In the real world, any measurement and observation will only provide us with some of these values (for instance, only in the proximity of detection instruments or speeding cameras). Typically, the missing data are provided (in an approximate way, inevitably) by surrogate numerical models, called *initialisation models*. This is a rather complicated story that we will not investigate here; we shall, nevertheless, describe a few examples when later dealing with more specific situations.

1.2   Approximate in Order to Solve

Let us go back to the model. If we have done the job properly, we should have managed to find the relationships between the unknowns (speed of the current, height of the water) and the data (shape of the river, roughness of the bed surface, upstream flow rate, status at time zero), thanks to mathematical laws (the differential equations) that express the fundamental and universal physical principles that represent the process under exam (the water flow in a basin).

Often (actually, almost always) this lands us on an extremely complex mathematical problem, much different from those we have seen in school. This problem will be so complicated that it will not be possible to solve it by hand. We will therefore need to use a computer. Before that, though, we shall need to *approximate* our model, that is, turn it into a similar model that can be translated into an algorithm, hence solvable by computer. For this reason we call the latter a *numerical model.* Clearly we should make sure that the solution to the numerical model is very close to the one we might have found if we had been able to solve the original mathematical model.

Speaking in general, the overall number of unknown variables is called the *dimension* of the system. Numerical models, which a computer must be able to solve, have one feature that cannot be waived: they must have *finite dimension.* This means they must have a finite number of unknowns, and that the algorithm computing them must consist of finitely many steps. (This fact is not obvious. For instance, calculating the sum of the inverses of all integers squared from 1 onwards requires, in theory, infinitely many steps.)

The passage from the infinite dimension of the mathematical model to the finite dimension of the numerical model is typical of the entire process. How do we go about it? It is not simple, and there is no standard way to do it. In fact there is an entire branch of mathematics (called numerical mathematics, numerical analysis, or approximation theory) that develops and studies constructive procedures for the various types of physical problems. Let us discuss an example within the river picture.

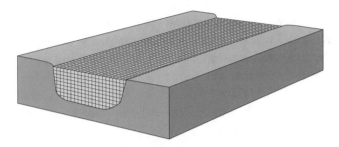

Fig. 1.1 The riverbed divided into a collection of tiny cubes of the same size

The mathematically exact solution should give the required values (for the speed etc.) at *each one* of the infinitely many points in space and time. We shall however content ourselves with finding the values at a number of selected points: the vertices (and perhaps also the centres) of a grid obtained dividing 3D space in cubes of *very small but finite* size (Fig. 1.1). The same should happen for time: we will find the values corresponding to finitely many instants separated by regular intervals.

Back to our example, let us take cubes with edges of 1 m and 10 minute intervals. Suppose the river is 1 km long, the river bed and banks are completely smooth and the basin's cross section is constant, say 10 m wide and 5 m deep on average (ok, no river is that regular, but we are simplifying, right?). If we intend to predict the surge over a 24 h period (from 12 pm today to 12 pm tomorrow) we will need to find the unknown values of $24 \times 6 = 144$ time instants (one hour is made of six 10-minute intervals), corresponding to $1000 \times 10 \times 5 = 50,000$ water cubes. Then on each cube we should solve the numerical model for the three components of the velocity (because at any point the velocity of a water particle is determined by its components along the three spatial directions), for the pressure and for the elevation (at least for the cubes on the bottom surface). I will spare you the calculations: just be aware that the final problem has 210,000 unknowns and must be solved 144 times. The numerical model has therefore dimension $210,000 \times 144 = 30,240,000$. This goes to show that a relatively simple situation may lead to models of whopping dimension.

1.3   How Many Models for One Problem? How Many Problems for a Single Model?

The chosen model has 1 m wide cubes, which might not be enough for an accurate forecast. We might need to take edges of 50 cm, and in case of a fast moving surge we might want to monitor the situation every minute rather than every ten. The kind of approximation will not be made empirically, but on the basis of rigorous mathematical arguments. Put differently, we have to ensure that our numerical model is able to provide accurate solutions that allow for a faithful representation of what will happen in reality. No surprise then that there may exist *several models* to describe the *same physical process*. The construction of a model depends on the *quantity of knowledge* over the phenomenon we wish to incorporate. In other words it depends on the degree of simplification we deem acceptable for our ends. Modelling is actually synonymous to approximating: often, reality is far more complex than our capacity to represent it.

On the other hand it may happen that a *single model* is apt to represent *distinct physical processes*. As surprising as it may seem, the equations describing the water surge in a river can also describe the evolution of the weather in a certain region, and with a little imagination (this is where abstraction comes into play!) they help to quantify a hedge fund's financial risk. Needless to say, the data, and even more the variables representing the model's solutions, will have a different meaning from those of the flood model. The common thread is the model's *mathematical structure*. This unifying capacity makes the approach via models extremely versatile, general and powerful.

1.4   The Phases of a Model

To build a model therefore means to complete a process consisting of many phases, which we may summarise as follows:

- understand the most relevant aspects of the concrete physical problem (in the example, the speed of water, its pressure, the height of the surge at each point of the basin, the expected time of a prediction);
- determine the essential data (the river's shape, the basin's smoothness, the initial flow rate, the unknown variables' values at time zero);
- translate this collection of information into a system of equations in the unknown quantities—the solutions, which are interrelated and depend on the data: this is precisely the mathematical model;
- transform the mathematical model into an approximate numerical model;
- build an algorithm to solve the numerical model, that is a finite number of steps, each of which consists of unambiguous mathematical procedures implementable on a computer;
- let the computer execute the algorithm, using a programming language (Matlab, Fortran, C++, Python, Java etc.);

- verify that the solutions provided by the computer agree with the observations of the initial problem: this phase is called *validation* and is essential to guarantee we have operated properly.

In the ensuing chapters we shall examine several models in action, on problems that display a rather different nature.

2

Weather Forecast Models

Abstract Predicting tomorrow's weather is a mathematical problem. The main quantities at stake are the air density, its temperature, pressure and speed. The current meteorological models are increasingly reliable, because of the advancements in atmospheric physics and the growing computational power of supercomputers.

If we did not have a model to predict the weather maybe the course of history would have taken a different turn. The decision to land in Normandy on that particular day (D-Day, 6th of June 1944) was taken based on the first mathematical model capable of making forecasts with a certain accuracy.

The weather has always played a key role in all human activities. Not only regarding our leisure (shall we organise a picnic in the countryside next Sunday?) or tourism (is it likely to rain at a given seaside resort at the end of July?), but also for organising the countless jobs that take place

© The Author(s), under exclusive license to Springer Nature
Switzerland AG 2022
A. Quarteroni, *Modeling Reality with Mathematics*,
https://doi.org/10.1007/978-3-030-96162-6_2

outdoors. Just think about agriculture, for which it is fundamental to decide when to do certain jobs like sowing and harvesting, farming, planning when herds go out grazing, or to plan transportation, be it of people or goods, by land, sea or air. Weather forecasts are helpful in a number of other potentially dangerous situations like predicting the chances of snow avalanches, floods or tropical cyclones.

Indeed, atmospheric phenomena have always been considered the paradigm of unpredictability. Nowadays, even technically advanced societies can suffer severe damages caused by extreme meteorological events. The impact is even more critical on lesser developed countries, where the quantity and nature of rainfall is crucial for the actual survival of the population. Over the last decades, moreover, forecasting the weather has become increasingly tied to the problems of anticipating *climate change* (that is, the trends in air and sea average temperatures and rainfall over decades if not centuries) and predicting air pollution levels.

In this chapter we will present a brief history of the mathematical models for weather forecasting, and the numerical models developed in the twentieth century with the aim of producing effective and accurate predictions, based on a coherent mathematical description of the atmosphere.

2.1   A Model Based on ... Thin Air

Addressing the weather forecast problem rigorously is not easy, as attested by the fact that the first comprehensive mathematical description only goes back to the start of the twentieth century. In 1904 the Norwegian mathematical physicist Vilhelm Bjerknes (1862–1951) suggested that we describe the motion of the atmosphere by modifying the equations governing a special class of gases, called ideal gases for their behaviour and considered *ideal* from many points of view [1]. We could say that modern meteorology was born at that moment. Bjerknes is the founder of the *Bergen School of Meteorology*, named after the town where he worked (is it not interesting that modern weather forecasting was born in a very rainy town?)

How can atmospheric air circulation be possibly modelled? How can we capture winds and clouds in mathematical equations? To begin with, we must understand what we should focus on. We are certainly interested in air and water in all their various manifestations: clouds, oceans, rivers, snow, ice, rain and wind. Notice that all these are fluid objects: they occupy the available space in a homogeneous and continuous way, without interruptions or empty parts. We must in fact begin from the space these elements occupy.

Let us consider the atmosphere, the casing of gases enclosing our planet that is held in place by the earth's gravity. We can divide it in varying layers distinguished by their composition: the troposphere (the closest layer to us, in direct contact with the earth's crust), the stratosphere, the mesosphere, the thermosphere, the ionosphere and the exosphere. The troposphere reaches the altitude of 12 km above sea level (to have an idea, airliners typically cruise between 10,000 and 12,000 m). The atmosphere's stratification is determined by the phenomenon known as vertical thermal inversion: in the troposphere the temperature decreases with the altitude, by about 6.5 °C every 1000 m, until we reach the layer's outer boundary where it begins to increase. In the stratosphere, thermosphere and exosphere the temperature increases with the altitude because of the direct absorption of the solar radiation. The transition between neighbouring spherical strata occurs across a discontinuity surface called *pause*.

To create forecasting models one concentrates on the troposphere and the lower stratosphere (13–15 km), for it is at these altitudes that high-level clouds (cirrus and cumulonimbus clouds) form.

2.2   The Physical Quantities Relevant to Meteorology

Weather forecasting involves several physical quantities. Just to mention a few, air density and pressure, wind speed, gravitational pull, heat exchanges between the air and the oceans, orography (the features of the earth surface: plains, hills, mountains, deserts, oceans, glaciers, forests, tundras etc.). Some of these will feed the model in the form of data, that is, known quantities (for instance the topographic relief, gravity, or the planet's angular acceleration). Others will be unknowns representing the model's solutions (most notably, air pressure, temperature and wind speed).

As we have seen in the previous chapter (recall the river current), we shall try to construct a model starting from the basic principles of physics: the conservation laws of mass and force. We shall apply them to *infinitesimal fluid elements*, which we may imagine as small cubes piled on one another in long columns, from the base (the earth's crust) to the highest altitude at which we wish to study the atmospheric motion (the stratosphere's lower boundary, say). All in all we will study hypothetical cubes made of, erm, thin air.

Let us begin from the balance equations: the mass of the fluid must be preserved, and the forces acting on the fluid should be in equilibrium. These laws must hold in each cube. After, we apply the mathematical procedure called *limit*, so we make the cubes smaller and smaller and find equations that we can assume hold at all points of the physical space and at all times: from the initial instant (when the model starts) to the final instant, the maximum time we wish to cover with the forecast.

This process is far from elementary, and we shall definitely not give the details here. Instead, we shall briefly describe the balance equations that need to be imposed, and discuss the type of equations that arise and their variables, in other words the unknown quantities.

2.3 Physics Comes to the Rescue

First of all, let us summon the principle of classical mechanics (perhaps better known in the formulation for chemical reactions due to Antoine-Laurent de Lavoisier) whereby *"Nothing is lost, nothing is created, everything is transformed"*. We apply it in our situation to every infinitesimal volume. At each instant the mass inside a cube equals the initial mass present, plus the ingoing mass flux, minus the outgoing flux (these fluxes are computed across the walls, the lateral surfaces of each cube). For example, if at the initial time the cube contains a million air particles and during one second 50,000 have entered and 100,000 have exited, then after one second there will be 950,000 particles. But how can we know how many go in and out? These are unknown quantities. It is reasonable to assume that the flux of particles through the cube walls depends not only on the speed of the air but also on its density. If the speed is constant, in fact, then the thinner (less dense) the air is, the greater the flux will be. Speed and density will be our first unknowns: the balance of the mass thus translates into an equation depending on the speed and the density. Starting with the infinitesimal volumes, the usual limiting process mentioned above produces an equation containing not just our unknown quantities but also an indication of how they change, instant by instant: these are the quantities' derivatives. (To be absolutely precise, the unknowns are the density and the *flow rate of the mass*, namely the mass at each instant, which is obtained by multiplying the speed and the density).

So now we have an equation in two unknowns. This is not enough to solve the problem, and we must have another equation. To find it we impose another physical law, *Newton's second law of motion*, according to which at any point in space and time the mass of fluid times its acceleration equals the net force acting on the fluid.

The net force is the sum of two kinds of forces: volumetric forces and surface forces. The former concern the entire mass contained in our cube: this includes gravity, the Coriolis force (due to the earth's rotation) and also the cohesive attraction between molecules. The nature of molecular cohesion depends on the specific material under exam (a gaseous fluid in our case) and is determined through suitable experiments. Mathematically speaking, they are expressed by *constitutive equations*, relationships among quantities such as the stress forces applied to the material and the deformations they generate. Surface forces, instead, are exerted on the walls of the air cube only. Putting everything together we end up with an equation depending on several quantities: acceleration, the rate of change of pressure between arbitrarily close points, the earth's gravitational potential, plus other more technical terms (more precisely: one term which represents the dissipation due to atmospheric turbulence and one accounting for the various heat sources that feed energy into the cube of fluid).

In order to write down this equation, though, a new variable was introduced: the *pressure*. So here we go again: to solve the problem we need yet another equation. Normally this is a suitable *equation of state*, an algebraic relation between density and pressure. But there is a but. That relationship is expressed by a term proportional to the fluid's temperature, so we are back to the start. Another variable appears, the *temperature*, which requires one equation more. So we impose the condition that the fluid is in thermal equilibrium (thermal balance equation) as prescribed by the *first law of thermodynamics*. And that is it, at long last!

Gathering all the equations found so far we have a *system* with several unknowns.

Conservation of mass:

$$\frac{\partial \overset{\frown}{\rho}}{\partial t} + \overset{\frown}{\vec{\nabla}} \cdot \left(\rho \vec{v} \right) = 0$$

where $\overset{\frown}{\rho}$ is the density and $\overset{\frown}{\vec{\nabla}}$ is the spatial divergence.

Newton's second law of motion:

$$\frac{\partial \vec{v}}{\partial t} + \vec{v} \cdot \vec{\nabla} \vec{v} + 2\, \overset{\frown}{\vec{\omega}} \times \vec{v} + \frac{1}{\rho} \vec{\nabla} \overset{\frown}{p} = -\vec{\nabla} \underset{\smile}{\phi} + \overset{\frown}{\vec{F}}$$

where $\overset{\frown}{\vec{\omega}}$ is the angular velocity of the non-inertial reference frame, $\overset{\frown}{p}$ is the pressure, $\overset{\frown}{\vec{F}}$ are the other forces acting on the fluid, and $\underset{\smile}{\phi}$ is the (Earth) gravitational potential energy.

Equation of state:

$$p = \overset{\frown}{R}\, \underset{\smile}{T}\, \rho$$

where $\overset{\frown}{R}$ is the universal gas constant and $\underset{\smile}{T}$ is the temperature.

Thermal balance equation:

$$\overset{\frown}{c}_v \left(\frac{\partial T}{\partial t} + \vec{v} \cdot \vec{\nabla} T \right) + p\vec{\nabla} \cdot \vec{v} = Q$$

where $\overset{\frown}{c}_v$ is the specific heat capacity at constant volume.

2.4   The Initial Data and the Boundary Data

This is a monster system, one that no mathematician would ever be able to solve explicitly and provide a clear and definite expression for the unknown variables. There is a glimmer of hope though: under certain conditions on the problem's data, it can be proved that, theoretically, there is a solution (and that it is unique: there cannot be others—at least within a short time frame). These conditions are about the *initial data*, meaning the values of the dynamical variables, namely the speed, temperature and density of the air at the initial time of the forecast (this is the *initialisation* mentioned in Chap. 1), and also the *boundary data*, those at the frontier of the region we are examining. The equations subsuming the latter are called *boundary conditions*.

Right, but where is this *boundary*? Or rather, how big is the region we are working in? Before we attempt to answer that let us note there are two different types of weather forecasting models. There are *global* models (*continental*, or *world-wide*) and *local* models (with regional reach, aka *limited area models*). The latter usually cover a country, like Italy, or specific regions, such as Sicily. For LAMs the boundary is the entire perimeter of Italy or Sicily. The boundary values are provided directly by the global models (like the continental one for Europe), that should in principle compute the unknown variables on the boundary of any sub-region of the planet. The global planetary model, on the contrary, has no boundaries: after all, the earth is (roughly) a sphere. In this case the boundary conditions subsume the spherical shape. If we started from any point on the surface of the earth and travelled along a meridian line or the parallel through that point, after a full circumnavigation we would return to the initial point, and clearly we would find the same values for the pressure, the temperature etc. Furthermore, if we wanted to limit the simulation to an altitude of, say, 13 km at most, hence to a spherical shell contained in the stratosphere, under the simplest possible assumptions we could prescribe a uniform value for temperature, density and wind speed in the upper layer of the shell.

The above system is, from a strictly mathematical viewpoint, solvable once the initial data and boundary conditions are given. That said, in practice finding this solution is a massive endeavour. First of all, the initial dataset relative to the atmosphere status is available only at a relatively small number of points (those where the detectors are positioned), and they refer to physical variables that differ from one another and vary from point to point. Furthermore, they are affected by measuring errors that cannot be neglected. Secondly, a realistic description of any meteorological phenomenon cannot refrain from the atmospheric distribution of water vapour, its phase changes (from gas to liquid and vice versa) and the ensuing rainfall. All these aspects complicate a lot the task of making accurate, quantitative forecasts.

2.5 Numerical Models, from D-Day to von Neumann

Summarising, there is no hope to solve our system by hand. It therefore becomes inevitable to resort to a suitable numerical approximation, so to render the system translatable into an algorithm, and eventually solve it with a (powerful) computer.

The first attempt to tackle the numerical resolution of the equations of motion is due to the British scientist Lewis Fry Richardson (1881–1953). During the first half of the twentieth century Richardson managed to describe the main phases of weather forecasting based on a mathematical model and on the numerical approximation of the equations of motion. He also introduced new concepts and tools in many mathematical subjects like numerical analysis, linear algebra and fluid mechanics. For his contributions, nowadays considered classical results, the name Richardson is familiar to many mathematicians, although few are aware of the peculiar context (meteorology) in which his ideas came to fruition.

Richardson's pioneering effort, told in a 1922 book [2], culminated in the first concrete numerical solution of a system of equations governing the atmospheric motion over a region as wide as the entire Western Europe. The author himself did all computations by hand, over a number of years and often in near-fictional circumstances. During World War I Richardson, a conscientious objector on religious grounds, was a nurse on the French front. He used every free moment to wrap up a part of the massive amount of arithmetical computations required.

Unfortunately his work did not have any immediate practical fallout. Despite the impressive computing effort, his results produced a completely wrong prediction. On the other hand, his contributions laid the ground for modern weather forecasting. For the first time in history someone had analysed every component of a numerical model for atmospheric circulation, following a conceptual scheme that is not dissimilar to the one used at present. Furthermore, it was the first time that a problem with no analytical solution (that is, exact, explicitly representable on paper) had been tackled using the strategy of applying numerical techniques to a simplified situation. In the most visionary and renowned passage of his work, Richardson imagined a gigantic amphitheatre filled with tens of thousands of (human!) *calculators* performing in parallel (independently from one another) the arithmetical computations of his atmospheric model on different continents, with the aim of generating in real time a mathematically sound forecast based on the computing technology available at his time. A precursor, some might say, of today's parallel computing [3].

Decisive in making Richardson's vision concrete was the contribution of the heirs of the Bergen School, in particular that of the Swedish meteorologist Carl-Gustaf Rossby (1898–1957). After studying under Bjerknes, Rossby emigrated to the US in the 1920s. In America he held top positions at the US Whether Bureau, MIT and the University of Chicago. He contributed to the founding of the weather division working for civil aviation and the army during WWII. In some sense, the decision to land in Normandy exactly on D-Day (June 6, 1944) is also due to his work.

Rossby identified some of the characteristic features of large-scale atmospheric circulation, such as jet streams and what we now call Rossby waves [4]. He was also responsible for significantly simplifying the general equations of atmospheric motion [5]. The use of these simplified models was also key to the first forecast made by a computer [6], a result of the Princeton collaboration between John von Neumann and Jules Charney, a former student of Rossby in Chicago, in the late 1940s. With that system, the errors in the measurements needed to recover the problem's initial and boundary data had a smaller impact on the quality of numerical solutions.

In 1950 it became possible to predict the weather on a region almost as large as North America, using a simplified model describing the atmosphere as a single stratum of a uniform fluid. In order to forecast over the next 24 hours an equal amount of time was necessary on the only existing computer of the time, the ENIAC. Nonetheless, the work of Charney and von Neumann proved, for the first time, that a prediction based solely on a numerical model was able to achieve results both qualitatively and quantitatively not far from the forecast obtained by an experienced meteorologist using the same dataset.

2.6 Increasingly Sophisticated Models: Lorenz's Butterflies

With this background, and thanks to the advancements in computer science technology and mathematical modelling, the fifty years ensuing the first work of Charney and von Neumann witnessed a continuous improvement in forecasting as regards both accuracy and reliability. This is not the place for a detailed account, but if we wanted to identify a few key elements that prompted a major progress in weather forecast, apart from the obvious spectacular increase in computer performance, we should focus on these fundamental aspects: the use of high-precision numerical methods to approximate numerically the equations of motion; the advancement of data-assimilation techniques (to which we shall return); the systematic and increasingly pervasive use of satellite detection [7, 8].

Another essential contribution to making finer forecasts came about when we eventually understood better the peculiarities of *non-linear* and *chaotic* dynamical systems, such as those governing the atmosphere. The notion of a chaotic system, that later became so relevant and almost hip, was born out of the work of a meteorologist, Edward N. Lorenz (1917–2008) [9, 10]. By simplifying the equations of atmospheric motion Lorenz wrote down a small system of two equations (subsequently turned famous under its

creator's name) with the aim of verifying the possible instability of the atmosphere. Lorenz, more precisely, wanted to
study a precise phenomenon: that the atmosphere's dynamics may amplify an even very small uncertainty in the initial
data to the point of preventing any sensible prediction over
its future state. It is for this reason that a two-week weather
forecast, or longer, cannot be accurate.

As a matter of fact Lorenz was the first person, in 1962,
to analyse the so-called *butterfly effect*. An excerpt from a
paper published by the New York Academy of Sciences [11]
reads *One meteorologist remarked that if the theory were correct, one flap of a seagull's wings would be enough to alter the
course of the weather forever*. Lorenz discovered the effect
while observing that the tiniest change in the initial data of
his non-linear system would have produced a completely
different outcome. In later speeches and papers Lorenz used
the more elegant butterfly as a symbol, perhaps inspired by
the plot generated by a special instance of his system, the
so-called *Lorenz attractor*, that does indeed look like a butterfly (Fig. 2.1). The official birth date of the butterfly met-
aphor might be 1972, when Lorenz gave a talk in Brazil
entitled *Does the flap of a butterfly's wings in Brazil set off a
tornado in Texas?*

One merit of this kind of study, in the field of chaotic
dynamics, is to have highlighted the limitations of a purely
deterministic set-up for the weather forecasting problem,
thus paving the way for probabilistic techniques. Put differently, today we no longer say *tomorrow it will rain*. We
rather tell the odds of it raining. Predictions, whether global
or local [12], are now done in this way.

What is more, the detailed analysis of the phenomenon
whereby everything depends on the quality of the initial
dataset has stimulated the development of novel techniques

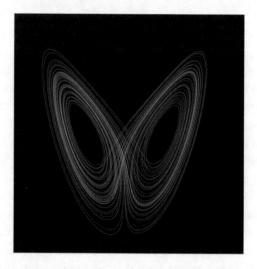

Fig. 2.1 Lorenz's butterfly-shaped diagram. Photo: zentilia/ Shutterstock

of *data assimilation* [13, 14]. These techniques allow to incorporate in the numerical model millions of single measurements made on a daily basis throughout the world using the most disparate means. In fact, even leaving aside the significant theoretical advances, there is no doubt that the better quality of weather forecasts is strongly related to the great improvement, both qualitative and quantitative, of the data available. Starting from the 1960s, in particular, besides the measuring stations on the surface (of which, paradoxically, there are fewer due to the high running costs), we also use satellite surveying systematically. These provide the bulk of the data used to initialise numerical models, nowadays.

2.7 Weather Forecasting Today

The impact of the scientific and technological advances we have discussed has been impressive. To get an idea of the degree of resolution and efficiency of the current models we might consider for instance some of the characteristics of the IFS, a global model of the European Centre for Medium-Range Weather Forecast (ECMWF) in Reading, UK. This prediction model, considered one of the best in the world, uses a grid with average horizontal spatial resolution of 22 km and 90 vertical levels. This means it employs cubes of fluid with a square base of 22 km per edge, and height of the order of 100 m, so it allows for the inclusion in the model of part of the stratosphere. The IFS can make 10-day forecasts on a modern parallel supercomputer in less than an hour, to which one must add a few hours for the complicated data-assimilation process. The prediction's accuracy is much better now compared to earlier models: just think that the average number of days covered by a reliable IFS forecast for Europe has passed from 5.5 in 1980 to 7.5 today. Even greater has been the impact of the new techniques over tropical zones and the southern hemisphere, where the scant network of measuring centres on the ground did not permit, in the past, reliable forecasts beyond one day. Today, instead, we have reached reliability levels comparable to the richest and most densely populated areas, due to the improved integration and assimilation of satellite observations.

Moreover, probabilistic predictions are nowadays a functional reality, one that provides a conceptually more accurate description of the evolution of a chaotic system such as the planet's atmosphere, and at the same time allows to quantify its margins of error in a given meteorological situation.

Among the other global models in use today we count the *United States Global Forecast System* (GFS), the *United Kingdom Met Office* (UK), the GME (Germany), the GEM (Canada), the JMA (Japan), the NAVGEM (US Navy), the SEMBAC (US) and the WMC (Russia). These models differ in several parameters, like the horizontal resolution, the orography involved, the mathematical model employed, the spatial numerical resolution and many more. In some cases we can only speculate, since often these models technical aspects have not been fully disclosed to users.

If one is interested in a smaller area (like a region), local-scale LAMs can be used. They possess a higher horizontal resolution than global models. Some LAMs have resolutions of the order of 1 km, which allows them to distinguish the forecasts of places 1 km apart. Moreover, they are suitable for short-term predictions: from a few hours (*nowcasting*, as opposed to *forecasting*) to two/three days tops.

To sum up, it is because of these spectacular achievements of mathematical models that, today, if we want to go on a Sunday outing we may look up the weather forecast and decide whether to head east, south, west or north to be sure we will find the sunniest meadow for a picnic or the windiest beach for windsurfing.

References

1. Bjerknes V. (1904), Das Problem der Wettervorhersage, betrachtet vom Standpunkte der Mechanik und der Physik, Meteorologische Zeitschrift, 21, pp. 1-7.
2. Richardson L.F. (1922), Weather Prediction by Numerical Process, Cambridge University Press, Cambridge.
3. Lynch P. (1992), Richardson's Barotropic Forecast: A Reappraisal, Bulletin of the American Meteorological Society, 73, pp. 35-47.

4. Rossby C.G. (1939), Relations Between Variations in the Intensity of the Zonal Circulation of the Atmosphere and the Displacements of the Semipermanent Centers of Action, Journal of Marine Research, 2, pp. 38-55.

5. Haurwitz J. (1940), The Motion of Atmospheric Disturbances on the Spherical Earth, Journal of Marine Research, 3, pp. 254-267.

6. Charney J.G., Fjrtoft R., von Neumann J. (1950), Numerical Integration of the Barotropic Vorticity Equation, Tellus, 2, pp. 237-254.

7. Robert A.J. (1966), The Integration of a Low Order Spectral Form of the Primitive Meteorological Equations, Journal of the Meteorological Society of Japan, 44, pp. 237-245.

8. Bourke W. (1972), An Efficient, One-level, Primitive Equation Spectral Model, Monthly Weather Review, 100, pp. 683-689.

9. Lorenz E. (1963), Deterministic Nonperiodic Flow, Journal of the Atmospheric Sciences, 20, pp. 130-141.

10. Lorenz E. (1969), The Predictability of a Flow Which Possesses Many Scales of Motion, Tellus, 21, pp. 289-307.

11. Lorenz E. (1963), The Predictability of Hydrodynamic Flow, Transactions of the New York Academy of Sciences, 25(4), pp. 409-432.

12. Molteni F., Buizza R., Palmer T.N., Petroliagis T. (1996), The ecmwf Ensemble Prediction System: Methodology and Validation, Quarterly Journal of the Royal Meteorological Society, 122, pp. 72-119.

13. Le Dimet, F.X., Talagrand O. (1986), Variational Algorithms for Analysis and Assimilation of Meteorological Observations: Theoretical Aspects, Tellus a, 38, pp. 97-110.

14. Rabier F., Thepaut J.F., Courtier P. (1998), Extended Assimilation and Forecast Experiments with a Four-Dimensional Variational Assimilation System, Quarterly Journal of the Royal Meteorological Society, 124, pp. 1-39.

3

Epidemics: The Mathematics of Contagion

Abstract Studying how a pathogen spreads among the population requires accurate mathematical models. The classical SIR epidemiological model divides the population in susceptibles, infected and recovered. Once the initial conditions are given, the numbers in each group vary in time under simple differential equations. A generalisation of the basic model is very well suited to describe the evolution of the current Covid-19 pandemic.

As we saw in the previous chapter, the first mathematical models (as we understand the notion today) were developed to study the weather, a phenomenon so ingrained in the day-to-day that it deserves our undivided attention. A few years after the birth of the first meteorological models mathematicians thought they should address another type of problems which, alas, has been with us since the dawn of time: the spread of infectious diseases through epidemics.

29

Epidemiological models, too, are a hundred years old by now, and may be thus considered *classics* in applied mathematics.

Before we examine the most famous among these models, called SIR, we must begin from a field that is only apparently distant: the ecological interactions between preys and predators, which we will see display behaviours similar to contagions.

3.1   Preys and Predators

Prey-predator interactions are as old as life on earth. Since the dawn of time there exist those who hunt and those who are hunted, in forests, steppes, seas and skies. The equilibrium of the species in a system depends on the ratio between the available resources and the number of consumers of those resources, hence it also depends on the ratio preys to predators. The whole picture has a complex dynamics. No surprise, then, that mathematicians have been keen on modelling this phenomenon for more than a century.

Whenever a mathematician is involved, everything is obviously always turned into equations. The most classical and renowned are the *Lotka-Volterra equations*, named after the mathematicians Alfred Lotka, who was born in the Ukraine and later became a US citizen, and Vito Volterra, from Italy.

Volterra got involved in the problem around 1925 by his son-in-law, the biologist and naturalist Umberto D'Ancona. While studying the Adriatic Sea fish fauna D'Ancona noticed that between 1915 and 1918 the sharp drop in fishing caused by World War I had altered the biological equilibria. Sharks, stingrays and other predatory species had increased their numbers at the expense of their preys, the fish that feed on plankton or small invertebrates (incidentally, these fish are what consumers most look for, so their diminished numbers had important economic consequences). Volterra, after examining the data, came up with a model based on two equations: one for the number of exemplars of the predatory species evolving as time goes by, the other providing the number of exemplars of preys. Clearly the two equations are tightly related (or *coupled*, as mathematicians say), because the two numbers vary according to the interactions between the two species.

In their simplest form the equations translate into mathematical terms several facts: predator y only eats prey x, the number of predator-prey encounters is proportional to xy, the variation of x is determined by the existing population and by the action of y, and conversely. In symbols:

$$
\begin{cases}
\underbrace{\dfrac{dx}{dt}}_{\substack{\text{rate of change in} \\ \text{the number of preys}}} = (A - By)\,\overbrace{x}^{\substack{\text{number of preys} \\ \text{present at time t}}} \\[3ex]
\qquad\qquad \text{positive parameters describing the} \\
\qquad\qquad \text{interaction between the two species} \\[2ex]
\underbrace{\dfrac{dy}{dt}}_{\substack{\text{rate of change in} \\ \text{the number of predators}}} = (Cx - D)\,\underbrace{y}_{\substack{\text{number of predators} \\ \text{present at time t}}}
\end{cases}
$$

So what happened during the war? When fishing reduces to almost nothing, predator fish have a larger number of prey available, they feast happily and their number grows. This obviously reduces the number of preys until the number of predators reaches a peak (let us remember this *peak*, we shall encounter it again in this chapter) and then starts to fall quickly. At this point prey fish can increase in number,

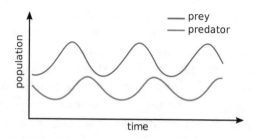

Fig. 3.1 The behaviour of the populations of prey and predators in time, according to the Lotka-Volterra model

but they have enemies, and so forth. What we have in practice is a cyclic (periodic) pattern in which the two curves of preys and predators intertwine and separate, in a life-and-death orchestrated dance (Fig. 3.1).

Needless to say this is a primitive model, which we may render more realistic by including terms that account for the season and climate conditions (animal reproduction is typically subject to fixed temporal cycles and is affected by temperature), the reproduction rates of the species involved, their longevity, the presence of external factors such as human intervention through fishing etc.

3.2   The Epidemiological Models

From a purely mathematical viewpoint, the study of the dynamics with which a pathogen (a virus, a bacterium or other) spreads among the population is not that different from the study of the interactions between preys and predators. We could think of pathogens as *predators* on the hunt for preys, meaning individuals to infect, and then proceed accordingly.

The earliest mathematical model in epidemiology was probably formulated over 250 years ago by Daniel Bernoulli (from a renowned family of mathematicians that vastly contributed to many areas), who wanted to endorse the cause for smallpox vaccination with his work. Bernoulli successfully demonstrated, mathematically, that if the entire French population got vaccinated, the average life expectancy would increase by more than three years. At the time life expectancy at birth was not high, and those extra years were a big change.

After the work of William Hamer and Ronald Ross in the early 1900s, the next cornerstone is 1927, when the Scots William Kermack and Anderson McKendrick proposed the famous model that bears their names. It was destined to become a reference work in the field of epidemiological modelling for years to come. It is a differential model of SIR type (in a short while we will see what this means), designed to explain the rapid growth and successive decrease in the number of infected people observed in certain epidemics, especially the plague and cholera. Since then the mathematical field of epidemiology has blossomed [1, 2]. One major step forward was passing from deterministic models to models that subsume casual fluctuations.

But one step at a time.

3.3   The Population's Critical Size: The Case of Measles

Before the role of pathogens in spreading infectious diseases was discovered, and way before the arrival of the first mathematical models, an apparently inexplicable phenomenon became manifest. Certain diseases (like the flu, measles or diphtheria) seemed to explode cyclically, alternating epidemic bursts and latent periods. Outbreaks appeared and disappeared periodically, especially in large cities. Why was that?

The discovery of the mechanism whereby epidemics seem to flare up and fizzle out is mostly a consequence of studies conducted on measles. Measles is a disease with which mankind has cohabited for millennia. Before the discovery of its vaccine it was endemic throughout the world and used to cause hundreds of thousands of deaths every year. (It has not been eradicated to the day, but the number of deaths has decreased a lot.)

In 1846 the Danish physician Peter Ludvig Panum observed a measles epidemic on the Faroe Islands directly. He was the first person to understand certain mechanisms governing the transmission, at a time when the role of pathogenic micro-organisms was still not known. In 1906 the English doctor William Hamer presented a striking result of his study: the interval between measles epidemics appeared to be constant. He collected the data in London, which at the time had a population of 5 million and was witnessing measles outbreaks every 18 months. Hamer also noticed that in smaller towns this phenomenon did not occur, and the disease's manifestations were more episodic.

The secret, as was discovered mid-century, lies in a number called *critical community size* (CCS). The critical community size is the smallest number of people in which the virus can persist endemically. The CCS varies with the disease and reflects its characteristics (transmission efficacy, virulence, permanent immunity of those who have recovered etc.). Measles has a CCS roughly equal to 500,000. In communities larger than half a million people (and in absence of a vaccine, naturally) the disease never disappears completely and returns periodically. Smaller communities, on the other hand, are reached sporadically, usually from outside, and after a while the infection dies out. Today the phenomenon is less accentuated in countries with strong global connections, but it still remains important in Africa, South America and parts of Asia [3].

3.4   A World of Susceptible Individuals

When dealing with an emerging virus (SARS, or the like) everything is more complicated. On one hand the virus's specifics are unknown: virologists do not know its genetic features, specialists in infectious diseases are unaware of its virulence. On the other hand the virus, being a newcomer, has the potential to infect the entire world population, since no human being has ever been in contact with the pathogen and did not have the chance to develop an immune response. We then say that the entire population is *susceptible*. This word refers to a person that has not contracted the disease, but might. Once a pathogen has found its first host (*patient zero*) and has infected them, this individual is potentially able to spread the disease according to the specifics of the virus (SARS infects through the airways, for HIV the transmission is of sexual nature). Susceptible individuals that come in contact with patient zero can get infected, and this is how the epidemic spreads.

The basic Kermack-McKendrick model starts by categorising the population in two groups: infected people (I) and susceptibles (S). Clearly, sooner or later some of the infected get better, and then pass to form a third category, the *recovered* (R). This group includes people who no longer transmit the contagion (so either they have healed completely, or they have died of it). This sort of model is called *compartmental* and is labelled by the acronym SIR.

Kermack and McKendrick introduced a fundamental parameter, known as the basic reproduction number R_0, that expresses the average number of susceptibles one individual might infect in the first phase of the contagion. The larger R_0 is, the more virulent the epidemic. The reproduction number of measles, for instance, is thought to be around 15. That is a very large number: an infected person will pass the virus to 15 others, on average, if none are vaccinated. For comparison, smallpox has an R_0 roughly equal to 7, for mumps R_0 is about 10, for chickenpox 8.5. But we need to be careful: we are talking about average values, computed over very large populations. In reality there are many infected people who do not infect anybody else, and also few so-called superspreaders. As regards SARS-COV-2, the coronavirus that was detected in China in 2019 and then infected the world over, the estimates vary a lot with the place and the moment. In Italy, for example, it is believed that R_0 is close to 2.5. This seems a low number compared to other viruses, but it is still very bad news. Just think that the R_0 of the Spanish Flu, that between 1918 and 1920 infected 500 million people and caused tens of millions of deaths, has been estimated, retrospectively, to be about 2.1.

As a matter of fact this is evident also mathematically. An epidemic with $R_0 = 2$ that is left to spread without countermeasures would lead to catastrophe. Starting from patient zero, we would then have 2, 4, 8, 16 infected people (remember these are averages), so 2^n infections after n iterations. The growth curve of infections would be exponential (Fig. 3.2). Although this model is simplistic, as we shall see in Fig. 3.4 it is reflected in the real data.

A dynamics of this kind can, without any intervention, lead to a massive percentage of infections (40–80%, depending on the pathogen), with unsustainable social costs.

We may ask why we do not reach 100%, given that the growth is exponential. Luckily enough, there are natural obstacles to the spread of an epidemic, like the so-called *herd immunity*. This term refers to the phenomenon whereby the healed and those that are immune for whatever reason, once they reach a certain critical number, start

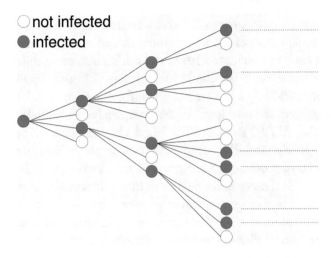

○ not infected
● infected

Fig. 3.2 The spread of the contagion for an epidemic with $R_0 = 2$

protecting the rest of the susceptible population, because they act as spacers. Moreover, there exist random variables (in this case favourable ones) that fight the spread of the virus.

Clearly, as the contagion progresses, the introduction of containment measures (also called NPIs, for non-pharmaceutical interventions) cause the number R_0 to decrease from its initial value, and we speak about the *effective reproduction number R_t*.

The critical value of R_t is 1: below this threshold every infected person infects on average less than one other individual, and the epidemic will eventually die out. When $R_t = 0.5$ for example, after n steps the average number of infected individuals is $1/2^n$, a number that becomes increasingly smaller as *n* grows. So if we want to contain an epidemic we should make sure R_t stays below that crucial value.

If there is a vaccine, to ensure the epidemic will extinguish itself we must vaccinate a fraction of the population larger than or equal to $(1 - 1/R_0)$. By putting in this formula specific values of R_0, we conclude that to eradicate measles we need to vaccinate 95% of the world population (and we are quite far from that), for poliomyelitis and smallpox about 85% (we are almost there for the former, whereas smallpox is considered to be completely eradicated), for SARS-COV-2 around 60%. In the absence of a vaccine we must rely on NPIs, which include the use of face masks, social distancing, shielding and so on. A quick calculation tells that if every individual came into contact with no more than 0.6 strangers on average, the Covid-19 contagion would stop. It is for this reason that one resorts to quarantines, social distancing, contact-tracing etc.

3.5   The Equations of the Contagion

Let us now see how one gets to the equations of an epidemiological model. For the easiest model we need a few simplifying assumptions. The first is called *homogeneous mixing*: every individual has the same odds of infecting any other person, irrespective of their previous contacts. It is obviously a rather unlikely hypothesis, since we all have more frequent contacts with family members, colleagues and friends, and we meet less frequently whoever does not live nearby or associates with other groups. Secondly, in the simple model we assume that the incubation period (the time between the infection and the appearance of the symptoms) and the course of the disease (the period between the first symptoms and recovery, or death) are constant. To make the model more realistic we should consider on one hand *heterogeneous mixing*, and on the other also contemplate the possibility that infected people are prevented from mingling at different rates, as a consequence of full recovery, immunity acquisition, isolation or death.

Let us stick with the simple situation. Susceptible individuals S that move out of the infected compartment I will widen the compartment of the recovered R, according to the pattern $S \to I \to R$. The probability of transition $S \to I$ is related to the number of contacts between one susceptible and the whole infected community. The same reasoning applies to the transition from I to R. The model should then contemplate the average times spent in phases S and I.

Let us indicate by s, i and r the relative quantities of people in each compartment, and by N the population's size. Then $s = \dfrac{S}{N}$, $i = \dfrac{I}{N}$ and $r = \dfrac{R}{N}$. Under these assumptions we deduce that the three quantities are related by the following equations:

$$\frac{ds}{dt} = -\beta s i$$

$$\frac{di}{dt} = \beta s i - \gamma i$$

$$\frac{dr}{dt} = \gamma i$$

where ds/dt, di/dt, dr/dt indicate the rates of change, that is, the derivatives, of the quantities s, i, r over time. (Shortly we will see what β and γ mean.)

To the above equations we must add the initial conditions. We should, in other words, establish the starting values s_0, i_0 and r_0 of the three quantities, those defining the situation in the population at the beginning of the period considered.

The values s_0, i_0, r_0 are positive or zero. Moreover, because of how s, i, r have been defined, we have $s_0 + i_0 + r_0 = 1$, and a similar identity $s + i + r = 1$ holds at any time.

By convention, $1/\beta$ is the average time between successive contagions. In this way the coefficient β in the first two equations denotes the average number of contagions per unit of time. The term $-\beta si$ expresses the speed of transmission from compartment S to compartment I. We indicate by 1 the average time spent in compartment I. Recalling that R_0 was the average number of susceptibles an infected person can pass the virus to, we will have R_0 = (average contagions per unit of time) × (average infectious period) = β/γ.

How do we assign a value to β and γ? One possibility is to start from the experimental data coming from animal infections. This procedure though is rather difficult and inefficient in the case of new epidemics. What happens in practice is that one estimates with statistical methods two quantities related to the infectious, or communicability, period. One is the incubation period mentioned earlier, that is, the time between the contagion and the manifestation of the symptoms. The other is the serial interval, which refers to the time between the appearance of symptoms in successive cases (Fig. 3.3). In the early days of SARS-COV-2, for

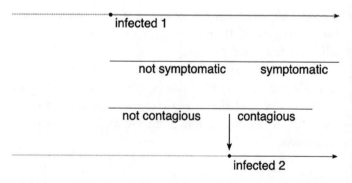

Fig. 3.3 A patient's symptomatic and contagious trend in time

example, Chinese scientists managed to estimate these two parameters quickly but only approximatively: an average incubation time of 5.2 days and an average serial interval of 7.5 days. A second possibility for gauging the parameters β, γ during an epidemic consists in comparing the model's results over a given time interval with the real data observed, and then choose the values and that minimise the difference. This procedure is called *model calibration*.

The presence of a time delay between the emergence of the infection in a new patient and the start of the communicability period prompts us to make a first generalisation of the SIR model, where we add a fourth compartment. This is the so-called SEIR model, with E indicating the exposed: infected individuals that are still not contagious. Several other generalisations are available. Figure 3.4, for instance, shows the SUIHTER model (named after the initials of its compartments) that has been successfully used for the simulation and forecast of the spread of COVID-19 in Italy starting from February 2020 [5,6].

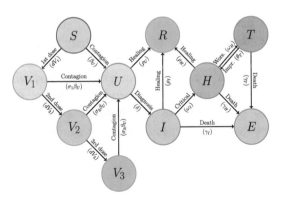

Fig. 3.4 The SUIHTER epidemiological model: S = Susceptibles, U = Undetected, I = Isolating at home, R = Recovered, H = Hospitalised, T = threat of life, E = expired

The main issue with these epidemiological models is their *deterministic* nature. The model only considers average values, and does not account for the fact that the contagion happens in a nonhomogeneous way, with random components. In practice a deterministic model such as SIR is only valid *asymptotically*, if we suppose there are infinitely many individuals (and it is for this reason that it works less badly with large populations).

A solution is to introduce *stochastic* equations, in which the unknowns s, i, r depend on random variables as well, to reflect the intrinsic uncertainty of the phenomenon modelled. But this complicates the calculations.

Other more sophisticated deterministic models subsume the population inhomogeneity in age and census, or in spatial distribution. If vaccines are already available, it becomes necessary to introduce an additional variable measuring the percentage of vaccinated population (or additional variables if vaccines are administered in several doses).

Also the computation of the CCS, which we discussed for measles, is based on compartmental epidemiological models derived from SIR. The more advanced models include seasonality, so for example there are less chances of contagion when schools are closed. A very much studied case is that of the African nation Niger, where the rainy season hampers movements (and hence the occasions of contagion) to the point that, during those months, the CCS of measles passes from 500,000 to 1.5 million [4].

3.6   The Peak, the Plateau, the Breakneck Slopes (and the Climb-Ups)

As we have observed, in the very first phase of the epidemic the models describe a contagion curve of exponential type. Even in absence of containment measures, the curve does not climb indefinitely (if this happened the entire population would go extinct). At a certain point the curve reaches a maximum, or peak, and then either goes back down or it stabilises on an endemic value. Containment measures are essentially in place to lower the peak value. The latter is sometimes less pronounced, looking more like a plateau than a proper peak. Once this value has been reached there is a slow descent in the number of new infections (Fig. 3.5).

The curve smoothes out according to the harshness and success of the containment measures, which can slow down and flatten the growth in contagions, thus attaining a peak

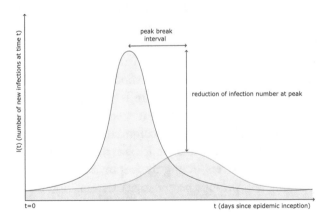

Fig. 3.5 The contagion curves with no intervention (blue) and containment measures (red). The integral between 0 and t, that is, the shaded area below each curve, provides the total number of people infected from day 0 to day t

that is lower and happens later. This slowdown is essential to allow the health system to prepare and be ready to treat a number of infected people not exceeding what the actual resources can take on. From an exquisitely mathematical point of view, pursuing that goal means introducing in the model further variables that represent the mitigation effects. The extra variables also act as *control parameters*, that is, parameters that can be tweaked in order to direct the system towards more acceptable results. (In mathematical jargon, one must ensure the solution to the SIR equations minimises the function counting to overall infection number.) See Fig. 3.6 for an example: the extent of the NPIs is described at the top using the colours adopted by Italian authorities (white-yellow-orange-red-black, from mildest to harshest). In this way, the scenarios analysed by mathematical models provide a vital support to the health authorities and civil defence. Such contributions are invaluable especially during the contagion's acute phase (where the contagion curve is exponential). But they can be very beneficial in later stages too. Often in fact there are backlashes in an epidemic, with ensuing new increases of the curve (albeit less violent) and successive adjustments. Let us not fool ourselves, though: very virulent epidemics are not easily tamed by mathematical models. Unpredictability lurks everywhere, and often there is no precise data available. Models allow to highlight trends as they happen, without pretending to give accurate numbers. Yet qualitative considerations can help politicians devise more efficient NPIs, raise awareness among the population about what is happening and prompt people to act responsibly.

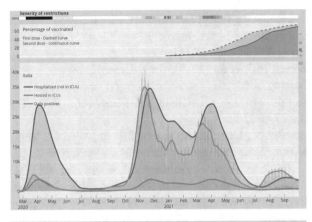

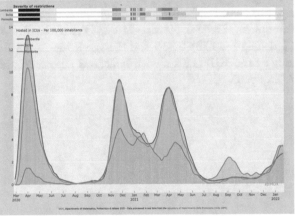

Fig. 3.6 Epidemic trend in Italy for the compartments hospitalised, daily positives, and hosted in ICUs (SUIHTER model)

References

1. Chen D., Moulin B., Wu J. (a cura di) (2015), Analyzing and Modeling Spatial and Temporal Dynamics of Infectious Diseases, Wiley, Hoboken, nj.
2. Pastore y Piontti A., Perra N., Rossi L., Samay N., Vespignani A. (2019), Charting the Next Pandemic: Modeling Infectious Disease Spreading in the Data Science Age, Springer, Cham.

3. Bartlett M.S. (1960), The Critical Community Size for Measles in the United States, Journal of the Royal Statistical Society, Series A (General), 123 (1), pp. 37-44.

4. Ferrari M.J. et al. (2010), Rural-Urban Gradient in Seasonal Forcing of Measles Transmission in Niger, Proceedings of the Royal Society B: Biological Sciences, 277 (1695), pp. 2775-2782.

5. Parolini N., Dede' L., Antonietti P.F., Ardenghi G., Miglio E., Manzoni A., Pugliese A., Verani M., Quarteroni A. (2021), SUIHTER: A new mathematical model for COVID-19. Application to the analysis of the second epidemic outbreak in Italy. https://www.arxiv.org/abs/2101.03369. Proceedings of the Royal Society A, 477 (2253), https://doi.org/10.1098/rspa.2021.0027

6. Parolini N., Dede' L., Ardenghi G., Quarteroni A. (2022), Modelling the COVID-19 and the vaccination campaign in Italy by the SUIHTER model, Infectious Disease Modelling, 7 (2), pp. 45-63.

4

A Mathematical Heart

Abstract Modelling the circulation of blood is a fluid dynamics problem, made complicated by the elasticity of the arterial walls and the formation of turbulence at the arteries' bifurcations. Yet the most stimulating challenge is translating into equations the heart's behaviour. A complete mathematical model has been recently developed at Politecnico di Milano and is being used for diagnosing and treatment of cardiac dysfunctions.

Twenty-five-or-so years ago I met with a young doctor specialising in vascular diseases who wanted my advice on a physically-related matter regarding blood circulation. I was rather taken aback, because the subject was very far from my usual field of work, but I immediately realised the problem was fascinating to a mathematician as well.

How do you go about in such cases, when you have to face areas of knowledge that are far from your own expertise? The first question one should ask, in total honesty, is

© The Author(s), under exclusive license to Springer Nature
Switzerland AG 2022
A. Quarteroni, *Modeling Reality with Mathematics*,
https://doi.org/10.1007/978-3-030-96162-6_4

47

whether one can say something relevant on the matter. The person who asked for advice wants concrete answers, and ignorance is no excuse. One should therefore understand the physical and biological phenomena at the heart of the problem, and then turn them into a model that phrases them mathematically. Is the model capable of answering the precise question we were asked? And if so, is it possible, afterwards, to return from the model to the concrete situation?

In the case of blood circulation the answer to all above questions is a sound yes. If we think about it, there is a tight relationship between medicine and numerical sciences. If we look at physiological phenomena such as muscle contraction, respiration, or blood circulation, we soon realise how any action, voluntary or involuntary, is the result of opposing forces produced by an *engine* and regulated at various levels by sophisticated mechanisms. Medical science, after long observing the natural processes governing the human body, became concerned with discovering the causes of ailments and studying their prevention. It does so through models of healthy behaviours and the early identification of risk factors. For its part, today mathematics is able to produce models that translate physiological mechanisms into equations, in some cases simulate the evolution of diseases, analyse the processes the body uses to absorb drugs, and so on. As we shall see further on, mathematics has recently started to enter operating rooms, by helping surgeons prepare delicate interventions.

In this chapter we shall focus on the circulatory system which, besides creating exceptional endeavours for mathematics, has an enormous social impact. Vascular diseases, in fact, are the main cause of death in the western world, being responsible for roughly 31% of all deaths world-wide (the percentage is above 40% in Europe). In particular, ischaemic heart disease is the primary cause of death in Italy, representing 29% of the total. More than cancer. Those who survive a heart attack often become chronic patients. The disease changes the patient's way of life and is a big economic burden on society. In Italy the latest National Institute for Social Security estimates (INPS) quantify the direct costs in 16 billion euros per year, plus another 5 due to indirect costs related to productivity loss. Cardiovascular diseases represent 19% of the pension scheme's total budget.

We shall first briefly examine, also from a historical perspective, what we know about the vascular system. Then we will model it in physical-mathematical terms. We will begin with the arteries, then pass to the *engine*, the heart, of which my research team at Politecnico di Milano is trying to create a digital model, in a project called iHEART financed by the prestigious European Research Council.

4.1 How Does the Cardiovascular System Work? An Eternal Challenge for Philosophers, Doctors, and Mathematicians

Understanding what the heart's purpose is and how it works is a challenge that has fascinated humanity since the dawn of time. In the third century BCE Aristoteles believed blood vessels transported *vital heat* from the heart to the periphery. A little later Praxagoras of Cos naively understood the different role of arteries and veins, and conjectured that arteries transported air whereas veins carried blood. We have to wait until Galen (second century CE), the forefather of western medicine, before it was recognised that arteries carry blood, too.

Jumping forward 11 centuries, between 1487 and 1513 the great Leonardo da Vinci made his studies of human anatomy. He was fascinated by the *machine of perfections*, as he described the human body. Leonardo's anatomical drawings are the most extraordinary piece of work his times allowed for. He was the first to define, with great precision, the four cardiac chambers, thus distinguishing the ventricles from the atria (formerly, auricles) and accurately describing the heart's cycle. According to Leonardo, this cycle was caused by the atria's contraction upon the diastole of the ventricles, whereas the ventricles' systole coincided with the atria's refilling. He called them motions of the heart (*moti del core*).

Another big leap forward bring us to the seventeenth century, when William Harvey inaugurated modern vascular research in his treatise *Exercitatio anatomica de motu cardis et sanguinis animalibus* (Anatomical exercise on the motion of the heart and blood in living creatures), which contains the first-ever correct description of circulation. Thanks to the beating-heart vivisection of various animals Harvey saw that the cardiac valves in the veins were designed to open only when blood flowed towards the heart, and concluded that *blood is in motion, and it moves in a cycle*.

In the subsequent century the great Swiss mathematicians Euler and Daniel Bernoulli made decisive advancements in the fluid-dynamical study of blood. In 1730 Bernoulli, then professor of Mathematics and Anatomy in Basel, formulated, whilst studying blood pressure, the famous equation of living forces (*vis viva* in Latin). This equation establishes the relationship obeyed by the blood's pressure, density and velocity (more precisely: half the density times the velocity squared, plus the pressure, is constant). In 1775 Euler, in the paper *Principia pro motu sanguinis per arteria determinando* (Defining the principles for the motion of blood through arteries), wrote a system of differential equations (still fundamental and employed in various contexts, like the study of gases inside a pipe or even airplane design) describing the evolution of the mass flow rate and pressure in a cylindrical, straight ideal blood vessel. A generalisation of his equations represent today the basic tool for simulating the blood flow inside the vascular system's intricate network of arteries and veins.

In the nineteenth century, whilst examining the arterial flow, the French surgeon and physicist Jean Léonard Marie Poiseuille derived the first simplified mathematical model of a stationary fluid (not varying with time) inside a cylindrical pipe, a model that still bears his name. More or less around the same time the British polymath Thomas Young made a cardinal contribution to the study of the properties of arterial tissues and the nature of the elastic waves propagating through them.

Among the twentieth century contributors we mention the American physiologist Otto Frank, who put forward a circulatory model based on the similarities with electrical circuits, and the British scientist John Womersley, who in studying the blood flow found the non-stationary (varying in time) equivalent of the Poiseuille flux, and precisely described the pressure variations throughout the entire cardiac cycle. But perhaps the greatest turning point of the twentieth century occurred in the applications of all the accumulated knowledge: cardiac surgery, thanks to open-heart operations, transplants and bypasses, has saved the lives of countless people, who had no hope of surviving before its introduction.

4.2 The Models Today

The past three decades have witnessed a vigorous growth of mathematical models for the circulatory system. Today we can build a virtual (mathematical) world in which we can solve equations that reproduce with great authenticity and precision the complex mechanical and biochemical processes occurring in the arteries, veins, and even inside the heart, as we shall see shortly [1]. An important physical characteristic is that the arteries' walls are elastic, and deform to facilitate the passage of blood.

A numerical simulation is illustrated in Fig. 4.1. Arteries are made of three layers, called (from inside outwards) tunica intima, tunica media and tunica adventitia. Across the arterial walls and the blood flow there is a constant energy exchange that mathematical models nowadays can simulate. This allows, in particular, to see how blood interacts with the endothelial cells that coat the vessels and the heart's innermost tissue, and how this affects their

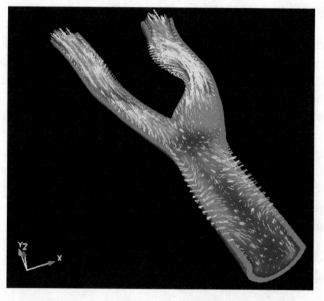

Fig. 4.1 Mathematical simulation of an artery's deformation

direction, deformation and possible damages. This is important also in view of understanding how degenerative processes arise, like those creating obstructions or the formation of plaques.

Furthermore, the blood flow equations consent to describe the transport, diffusion and absorption of several chemical components (like oxygen, lipids and drugs) in the various layers of the arterial wall, and ultimately allow to understand whether our tissues are properly nourished.

More generally, today's models and simulations can reconstruct a number of anomalous behaviours displayed by the blood flow, which are possible contributing factors to the start of a pathology. An important case, just as an example, are the vortices occurring past the carotid bifurcation (Fig. 4.2). The two carotids (left and right) are arteries that originate from the aorta immediately after the latter exits the heart, at the top of the aortic arch. Inside the neck each carotid splits into two branches, one of which brings

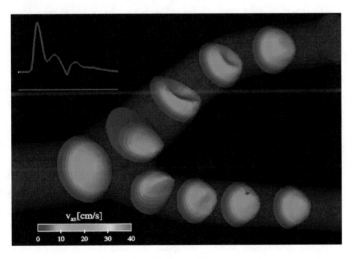

Fig. 4.2   Blood pulse inside the carotid

blood directly to the brain. It is here that the vortices occur. The problem is very general: vortices happen in vessels with large bends (the aortic arch for instance, or the coronaries) or whenever the pressure the blood exerts on the wall jumps in the fraction of a second passing between the systole (the heart's contraction) and the diastole (the dilation). Nowadays, also thanks to mathematical models, we begin to understand in detail phenomena like haemodynamics at a local level, the effects a modification in the walls has on blood flow, or the medium/long-term gradual adaptation of the whole system after a surgery (for instance after the removal of plaques).

Another case where mathematical models have made massive advancements, with useful applications, is coronaries. Coronaries draw blood from the first aortic tract, just outside the heart, and they convey it back to the heart or better, to the cardiac muscle, thus guaranteeing myocardial cells are nourished (the myocardium is the heart's muscular tissue).

Unfortunately, the coronaries have the tendency to occlude and hence deprive the myocardium of the necessary irrigation (doctors call it perfusion), which in the worst cases leads to a heart attack. In the majority of cases surgery is imperative to restore the flow, and this can happen in many ways: with a bypass, an angioplasty or by placing a stent.

In order to create a bypass one uses a portion of one of the patient's healthy arteries (or veins) to create an alternative route for blood. The deviation is sown on the vessel before and after the obstruction. There are many ways for doing this, and we may ask what will be the optimal way, the one benefitting the patient most. Obviously the concept of optimality is very subjective. Can mathematics help in this respect?

Despite this kind of surgery has become a routine, each year 8% of patients with a bypass implant risk a new occlusion. Moreover, after 10 years from the first operation a significant percentage must undergo surgery again (10–15% of arterial bypasses and 50% of venous ones; the latter grows to 85% after 15 years). Performing surgery a second time involves a high risk of complications, so one should be very careful to avoid problems after the first operation. In this respect, the simulation of the circulation in a coronary bypass, especially downstream from the reattachment point, can make us understand how much the arterial morphology affects the flow and hence the post-op evolution.

4.3   Mathematics in the Operating Room

Let us return to the model's application. A procedure less invasive than the coronary bypass seen above consists in the intravenous introduction of a stent. A stent is a microstructure made of metallic threads interwoven into a suitable shape. It is inserted closed, and then it is made to expand around the obstruction until the artery returns to its original diameter. This kind of device typically stays in place forever.

The implant of a stent is a much less invasive and onerous operation than a bypass, apart from being cheaper economically. Inserting the device in a vessel (Fig. 4.3), whether in a coronary, a carotid or another artery, changes the wall's stiffness and elastic properties. Therefore the treated part will, after the operation, react in a completely different way to the passage of the blood pumped by the heart. The stiffness in particular will increase. This causes one component of the propagating wave to be reflected and slowed down in

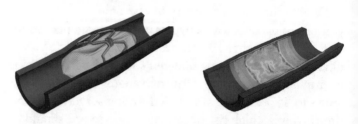

Fig. 4.3 Mathematical simulation of the effects of a stent [insertion] on the elasticity and stiffness properties of the arterial wall

the proximal area (near the heart), whereas it gets accelerated in the distal area (towards the periphery, far from the heart). Sometimes this generates a significant variation of the force the blood pressure exerts on the arterial wall. Mathematical models take this phenomenon in account and are useful in the process of designing more efficient stents.

Another source of problems is the fact that devices interact with the cells of the vessels' walls they are in direct contact with. Metals such as iron, nickel etc., constituting certain stent types, can interact with the cells of the tunica media and intima, thus causing an inflammatory response. In turn, that may trigger a rampant proliferation of smooth-muscle cells inside the tunica media and a reduction of the lumen (the hollow part of the vessel in which the blood flows). To counter this phenomenon, research has devised drug-eluting stents, which are micro-coated by a special material capable of storing and slowly releasing an anti-inflammatory active principle. Tiny holes can be made in a stent's fibres and then filled with layers of different substances. To that end, mathematical modelling and computer simulations allow to assess the behaviour of several configurations (Fig. 4.4), both quickly and in a much cheaper way compared with traditional testing [2, 3].

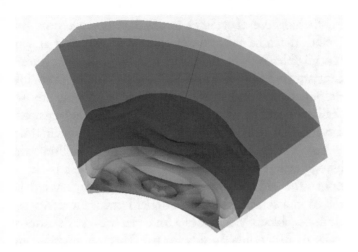

Fig. 4.4 Drug-eluting stent simulation

4.4 The Blood's Equations

Blood, in the eyes of physics, is not even a fluid, but a suspension of solid particles (white cells, red cells and platelets) in a fluid substance called *plasma*. In larger arteries (of diameter exceeding 2 mm-like epicardial coronaries and carotids) though, the behaviour of blood is completely similar to that of a homogeneous fluid, and therefore we shall treat is as such.

The model employed in this situation is based on the celebrated Navier-Stokes equations, which owe their name to the French physicist Claude-Louis Navier (1785–1836) and the Irish physicist George Gabriel Stokes (1819–1903). One of the Navier-Stokes equations rephrases Newton's second law: the mass of a fluid times the acceleration, at each point in the vessel and at each instant, equals the sum of all forces acting at that point. But while in Chap. 2 we applied the equations to the air (which is a fluid, let us not forget it) for the purpose of weather forecasting, here we need not include the force due to the earth rotation, which at present is negligible. We will, moreover, suppose the temperature is constant (in reality it is not, but it makes for an acceptable simplification), and so will the density. Consequently we shall not need the temperature equation, and the mass conservation law will not contain the density's variation in time.

The Navier-Stokes equations produce as solution the blood pressure and its velocity along the three spatial directions. The difficulty arises from the fact they should be solved in a small region (the arterial lumen, the cavity occupied by blood) that varies with time, because the arterial walls are distensible (luckily for us). Their contraction and relaxation, by the way, depend on the flow, so they represent further unknowns. To describe the walls' motion we will then need another equation, which will be coupled to the Navier-Stokes equations governing the motion of blood.

In formulating the new relations we will take inspiration from Newton's second law once again, but we will have to include the special structure of the arterial wall. As was mentioned, the wall is made of three layers separated by thin membranes, different in structure and mechanical behaviour. We therefore need another relation, called *constitutive equation*, for translating that particular structure in a system of relations between the forces acting on the walls and the deformations of the walls themselves.

There remains to describe the interaction of the blood flow with the arterial wall. We will do that using two *coupling* equations, expressing a kinematic condition (relative to the motion of blood) and a dynamical condition (relative to the force blood applies to the walls). The former translates the property that every blood particle that hits the wall will remain stuck to it, so from that moment it will move in sync with the wall (because blood is a viscous fluid). The dynamical equation, instead, states that the force exerted by blood on the wall is equal, but with opposite sign, to the force that the wall exerts on blood when deforming.

Summarising, the mathematical model will consist of: the Navier-Stokes equations for the fluid, the equations for wall motion, the constitutive equation and the coupling equations (kinematic and dynamical).

Navier-Stokes equations for the fluid (blood):

$$\rho \underbrace{\frac{\partial \vec{v}}{\partial t}}_{\substack{\text{acceleration} \\ \text{term}}} - \underbrace{\nu \, \Delta \vec{v}}_{\substack{\text{diffusion} \\ \text{term}}} + \underbrace{\rho \, \vec{v} \cdot \vec{\nabla} \vec{v}}_{\substack{\text{inertial} \\ \text{term}}} + \underbrace{\vec{\nabla} \, p}_{\substack{\text{pressure} \\ \text{gradient}}} = \vec{0}$$

fluid (blood) velocity   viscosity   density   pressure

$$\vec{\nabla} \cdot \vec{v} = 0$$

Elasto-dynamics equations for the arterial wall:

$$\underbrace{\frac{\partial^2 \vec{s}}{\partial t^2}}_{\substack{\text{acceleration} \\ \text{term}}} + \underbrace{\vec{\nabla}}_{\substack{\text{spatial} \\ \text{divergence}}} \cdot \left(\underbrace{\vec{\vec{\sigma}}(\vec{s})}_{\substack{\text{Cauchy stress} \\ \text{tensor}}} \right) = \vec{0}$$

wall displacement

Constitutive law:

$$\vec{\vec{\sigma}}(\vec{s}) = \vec{\vec{f}}\left(\vec{s}, \frac{\partial \vec{s}}{\partial t}, \lambda, \mu \right)$$

elastic coefficients of the arterial wall

Kinematic condition:

$$\vec{v} = \frac{\partial \vec{s}}{\partial t}$$

Dynamical condition:

unit vector orthogonal to the
epithelium (the lumen-artery interface)

$$v \frac{\partial \vec{v}}{\partial n} - p \vec{\vec{n}} = \vec{\vec{\sigma}}\left(\vec{s}\right) \cdot \vec{n}$$

4.5   At the Heart of the Problem

Until this point we have talked only about circulation. But what about the system's engine itself, the heart? Surely its modelling must be an even more complex endeavour.

Well, on the 1st of December 2017 we inaugurated an ambitious project iHEART, for *Integrated Heart*, at Politecnico di Milano. The goal is to realise a virtual mathematical model, made of a system of equations, capable of integrating every one of the processes of the cardiac function, and therefore able to reproduce the human heart's behaviour.

If one could build a virtual model capable of simulating all the functions and dysfunctions of the heart, there would be enormous rewards in terms of prevention and assistance to doctors. Even more if the study could be *personalised*, so to create a virtual heart for every single individual.

Our hearts beat because every second a spontaneous electrical impulse is generated in a specific region called the sino-atrial node, which is made of cells that excite involuntarily and thus make for a natural pacemaker of sorts. From there the sparkle produces an electric field propagating to the atria, then to the entire myocardium, thanks to a network of special fibres called Purkinje fibres; they work as a large network of fast lanes. This phenomenon is described by a series of equations, called the electrophysiology model.

Because of the electric impulse all cardiomyocites (the elementary cells of our heart) excite, depolarise and repolarise to give rise to a sequence of contractions and expansions. These induce, at the macroscopic level, the movement of the entire cardiac muscle, thus facilitating the ventricles' contraction and relaxation. The venous blood, full of carbon dioxide and other toxic waste, is sucked in the right atrium by the vena cava, and then passes in the right ventricle to be pumped through the pulmonary arteries to the lungs. Inside the lungs the venous blood releases its toxic components (eliminated through the respiration) and loads itself with oxygen. Through the pulmonary veins this enriched blood reaches the right atrium, then the right ventricle upon the atrium's relaxation. The successive contraction of the ventricle makes the blood overcome the aortic valve's resistance and get pumped in the ascending aorta, from where it reaches every corner of our body.

How can we represent all these processes mathematically? *Divide and conquer*: we begin by breaking down the problem in its main components. In the case at hand we will have: a) equations describing the electric potential created across cell membranes (the so-called transmembrane potential) and its propagation; b) equations describing the intensity of current produced in each cell by depolarisation and polarisation; c) equations describing the rate of contraction and relaxation of every single myofibril; d) mechanical equations allowing to simulate the motion of the whole myocardium, similar to those we met for the interaction between blood flow and arterial wall movement.

What is missing are the equations controlling how the fluid (blood) behaves inside atria and ventricles, and the

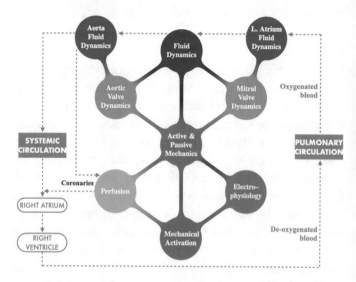

Fig. 4.5 A conceptual map that illustrates the different physical processes characterising the functioning of the left ventricle and their interactions

way our coronaries perfuse the myocardium. And that is not all. We must describe the dynamics of the four valves present in our hearts as well: the two that connect the upper and lower chambers (mitral and tricuspid), the pulmonary valve directing the venous blood to the lungs, and the aortic valve through which the arterial blood is pumped into the ascending aorta every second. There is no need to remark that all these models are interdependent, meaning that there are further equations that link the various unknowns together (Fig. 4.5).

The resulting system is the virtual model of the heart. It is made of 30 or so nonlinear and time-varying differential equations, whose number after the numerical approximations balloons to tens, or hundreds, of millions [4, 5]. To

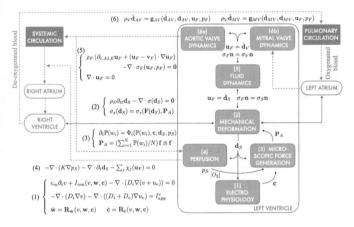

Fig. 4.6   A mathematical model of the heart's activity

solve them one needs a supercomputer capable of performing thousands of billions of algebraic operations per second (Fig. 4.6).

For it to function, this model requires data, and of varying nature. To begin with, we should start from clinical images (such as magnetic resonance, CT-scans) to reconstruct by geometrical techniques the shape of a specific patient's heart. But we will also need information on how the myocardial fibres are arranged, plus other parameters describing its electric conductivity. After a stroke, for example, there are scarred areas of the myocardium where the conductivity is, if not zero, much reduced.

As is easy to guess, these data are often hard to get hold of. It is for this reason that the creation of an integrated model of the human heart goes through the crucial collaboration with doctors.

From the mathematical point of view the heart poses the typical problems of living structures, which are further magnified by its intrinsic complexity. First and foremost is the lack of boundary conditions and, in general, the fact that not all relevant data are known or attainable. One must also represent non-standard objects (each one of us has their own heart and arteries), with nonrigid and geometrically complicated shapes. It comes down to the mathematician's creativity to complete the model in a manner that is not too invasive, that is, without assuming too many of the missing data nor oversimplifying. It is at this juncture that the expertise of medics, radiologists, cardiologists and other specialists becomes fundamental.

The heart is such a complex organ that we will never reach a completely exhaustive and precise description of it. Building a virtual, mathematical, heart, only made of equations, is a tremendous challenge; one that is worth accepting though, for our health would profit enormously from every small victory.

What should we expect in 10 or 20 years' time when doing a cardiac checkup? Will we have a personalised model of our own heart, that will allow for precise diagnoses and most of all enable the specialist to assess future risks?

We are on the way towards that scenario. At Johns Hopkins University in Baltimore, for instance, Professor Natalia Trayanova goes in the operating room to assist cardiologists in the difficult task of curing arrhythmias and ventricular tachycardias. She uses the simulations she made the day before with her fellow mathematicians and engineers, starting from the clinical images (MRIs and CT-scans) of the hearts of the patients that will undergo surgery.

The cases of collaboration between mathematicians and doctors, like this one, are more frequent than what we may think. Today mathematical simulations are employed to improve the treatment of patients in several areas, including oncology, pathologies of the cardiovascular system, the fitting of prostheses to replace damaged or compromised joints, and so forth.

The dream is to pass from a heart that pounds *because* of a maths test (who, as a student, did not experience this feeling?) to making the heart beat in a healthier way *thanks* to mathematics.

References

1. Formaggia L., Quarteroni A., Veneziani A., Eds. (2009), Cardiovascular Mathematics. Modeling and Simulation of the Circulatory System, Springer, Milano-New York.
2. Quarteroni A., Veneziani A., Zunino P. (2001), Mathematical and Numerical Modelling of Solute Dynamics in Blood Flow and Arterial Walls, siam Journal of Numerical Analysis, 39 (5), pp. 1488-1511.
3. Prosi M., Zunino P., Perktold K., Quarteroni A. (2005), Mathematical and Numerical Models for Transfer of Low-Density Lipoproteins Through the Arterial Walls: A New Methodology for the Model Set Up with Applications to the Study of Disturbed Lumenal Flow, Journal of Biomechanics, 38, pp. 903-917.
4. Quarteroni A., Dede' L., Manzoni A., Vergara C. (2019), Mathematical Modelling of the Human Cardiovascular System. Data, Numerical Approximation, Clinical Applications, Cambridge University Press, Cambridge.
5. Quarteroni A., Dede' L., Regazzoni F., (2022), Modeling the Cardiac Electromechanical Function: A Mathematical Journey, Bullettin of the American Mathematical Society, 59 (3), pp. 371-403.

5

Mathematics in the Wind

Abstract Optimising the shape of sails, minimising the drag of water waves and perfecting the aerodynamics of a hull can guarantee a decisive advantage at the finish line: Alinghi's triumphs in the America's Cup are also a victory for mathematics.

In the autumn of 2001 the President of École Polytechnique Fédérale de Lausanne (EPFL), where I taught, asked me to take part in a meeting. One of the attendees was rather unexpected: Russell Coutts, the legendary skipper who had just led New Zealand's *Black Magic* team to victory in the 29th and 30th editions of the *America's Cup*, the world's most prestigious sailing race. During that meeting we were told that Ernesto Bertarelli, a young successful entrepreneur and sailing enthusiast, had decided to create a Swiss team, captained by Coutts, to compete in the 31st edition of the *Cup*. The team would be called *Alinghi* (after the name of

© The Author(s), under exclusive license to Springer Nature Switzerland AG 2022
A. Quarteroni, *Modeling Reality with Mathematics*,
https://doi.org/10.1007/978-3-030-96162-6_5

the boat Bertarelli had received as a present from his father as a boy). The EPFL was asked to act as scientific consultant on the project. I remember the President bantering on how the media would cover the story (a team from a notoriously mountainous, and landlocked, country competing in the America's Cup …), and then telling me the EPFL would take on two tasks: the building materials (assigned to a colleague of mine) and the fluid dynamics design. The latter would be for me and my CMCS team (Mathematical Modelling and Scientific Computing) to solve.

No need to say I knew nothing about sailing. To prepare for the second meeting with Russell Coutts and Grant Simmer (the famous skipper of Australia II, the first non-American yacht to win the America's Cup after 135 years of uncontested US reign), I had to download from the web the 50 keywords of the sailing lexicon.

I could not possibly know that from that moment, and for the next 9 years, Alinghi would become a trusted travelling companion. It was an adrenaline-fuelled adventure, that led us to win the Vuitton Cup and then the 31st America's Cup in March 2003 in Auckland (beating Black Magic), the 32nd America's Cup in July 2007 in Valencia (defeating team Oracle), and to the February 2010 final, again in Valencia, that we lost to team Oracle.

I am sure you will be asking yourselves: what does mathematics have to do with the America's Cup? We will get there soon, but before let us look back at some history.

5.1 A Sports Trophy with a Glorious History

Apart from the Olympic Games, the America's Cup is the world's oldest sports competition. The first edition took place on 22 August 1851 at the Isle of Wight in the UK. The

British Royal Yacht Squadron, with 14 yachts, challenged the New York Yacht Club (NYYC), which was participating with one yacht only, a *schooner* called *America*. The Americans won, finishing 8 minutes ahead of the next yacht, the British Aurora, and were awarded the trophy that had been prepared to celebrate the first universal exposition in London.

The loss was a hard blow for the UK's invincible naval powerhouse, and the Brits called for a second match to get even. By regulation this had to be played in waters chosen by the NYYC. The Americans prevailed again, in one of an incredible string of triumphs: they were unbeaten in 25 events over 132 years, the longest winning streak in the history of any sport.

The turning point was 1983, when six challengers (called *syndicates*) signed up. To decide who would battle the Americans over the trophy, it was decided to hold a series of knock-out regattas, which became the *Louis Vuitton Cup*. Also participating in the 1983 edition, for the first time, was an Italian yacht, *Azzurra*. It ended up third and, most relevantly, had the merit of publicising the existence of the race among the Italian audience. If you happen to know an Italian named Azzurra born in the mid-80s, now you know why. The trophy was easily won by the Australian team Royal Perth Yacht Club, with Australia II (this yacht was equipped with technical innovations that were kept under wraps until the end). What is more, Australia II won the America's Cup, thus ending the US team's 132-year-old reign.

Research and technology stated to play a decisive role in that edition. The design of Australia II's winged bulb, for instance, was inspired by advanced aerodynamical notions, already exploited in aviation. The New Zealand yacht that came in second was the first 12-m class yacht with a fibreglass hull, rather than the usual aluminum.

In 1988 a New Zealand syndicate lodged a surprise challenge with a whopping 36-m yacht (a return to the yacht size of the early races). The challenger, the San Diego Yacht Club, exploited a hidden weak spot in the rules and built *Start and Stripes*, a small, 18-m catamaran, both agile and very fast, that crushed the reigning champions.

From 1988 to 2007 the rules changed to allow only 12-m yachts to race. In 1992, *America*[3] (read: America cubed) beat the Italian challenger *Il Moro di Venezia*. In 1995 the Team New Zealand syndicate won the race, with Russell Coutts as skipper of Black Magic. In 1999–2000, in the waters of Auckland, Team New Zealand prevailed again by defeating the Italian challenger Prada Challenge with *Luna Rossa*. The Italian yacht, helmed by the Neapolitan skipper Francesco de Angelis, had won the Louis Vuitton Cup by beating in the final race the US yacht America One, captained by Paul Cayard, formerly at the helm of Moro di Venezia.

5.2 The Swiss Outsider and the Mathematics of Sails

This is the moment when the history of the America's Cup crosses paths with my scientific account. In December 2001 I set up an EPFL team of three, who until that fateful 2nd of March, 2003 would stay in touch with Grant Simmer's design team and Russell Coutts's sailors. Videoconferences with the Alinghi team in Auckland (12 hours ahead) were held weekly at the crack of dawn for us, the end of the evening for them.

How does one, as a scientist, tackle a subject so distant from one's own personal history? The first thing is, clearly, understanding the problem, to decide whether one is able to take it on. "Understanding" here means examining in detail the physics and engineering aspects that are useful to the construction of the model. Initially the work is mainly theoretical, but one must then translate the knowledge acquired into the client's language, which also involves economic aspects and deadlines: compared to a curiosity-driven research, here there is the constraint of finite resources and, what is even more compelling, finite time.

The Alinghi job seemed really challenging: a gigantic object (24 tons in weight, almost 800 sq. m. of sails when fully open, a 25-m mast), with a complex geometry, subject to incredible forces and stresses. Two turbulent fluids are involved: air and water. The conditions of motion vary a lot: depending on the strength and direction of the wind, there could be aerodynamic lift effects similar to those on aeroplane wings, or drag as in parachutes, and so on. The extra-scientific constraints are – hard to conceive as it may be – even more severe. Large bags of money are at stake, and the line between victory and defeat is very, very thin. America's Cup races are ferociously competitive: even after a race that lasts hours, the two boats may cross the finish line a few centimetres apart. In contrast to what happens in industrial applications like aircraft design, where large security margins are required, here it is essential to reach extreme, razor-edge performances. Designers must push their creation's agility features to the limit, without exceeding the limitations of natural resilience.

An America's Cup monohull-type vessel (like those competing until the 32nd edition) is made of various components: in the water we have the hull, the keel, the bulb, plus other appendices such as winglets and the rudder; outside there are the mast and the sails—mainsail, genoa, spinnaker and gennaker (see Figs. 5.1 and 5.2). In the past there were very different shapes of hulls, keels and bulbs, but in the

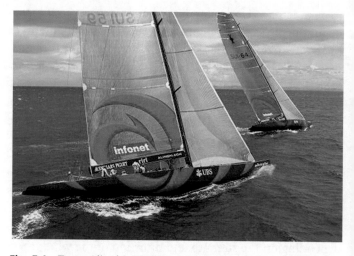

Fig. 5.1 Team Alinghi. 2003 America's Cup, Auckland, New Zealand. Picture: ChameleonsEye/Shutterstock

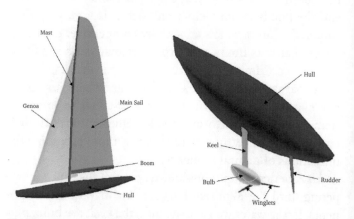

Fig. 5.2 Aerial and submerged components in a sailboat of America's Cup class

2000s (till 2007, the last year of monohull racing) a uniform standard was agreed upon. Hence it is the tiniest details that make a difference in terms of results. In 2003 Jerome Milgram, an MIT professor and a veteran consultant to America's Cup teams, said "America's Cup yachts require extreme precision in the design of the hull, the underwater parts and the sails. An innovative hull offering a 1% drag reduction can warrant a gain of 30 seconds at the finish line."

Let us come to the mathematics, and divide the problems in sub-problems. We begin with the hull. To optimise its performance we must solve the fluid dynamics equations around the whole boat keeping into account the regatta's countless conditions; the variations, for instance, of wind and sea waves, of the different sailing regimes (upwind, downwind), of the position and motion of the opponent vessel. We must also consider the dynamics of the interaction between fluid and structural components, meaning water and the submerged parts, as well as between air, sails and mast. Finally, we must model with great precision the shape and motion of the interface between water and air, the so-called free surface.

Let us introduce the *computational domain* Ω, the 3D region in which the equations must be solved. This domain consists of a parallelepiped of $300 \times 200 \times 180$ m. The lower part is occupied by water, the top part by air, and the boat sits in the middle. On the parallelepiped's (ideal, not physical) frontier we must impose boundary conditions reflecting the true, experimental boundary conditions needed to solve the differential problem.

The equations governing the flow around the boat are the dear old Navier-Stokes equations, here in the version for fluids with non-constant density (inhomogeneous fluids). In fact there are two fluids in the game: water (with a density of 1 g per cubic centimetre, that is 1000 kg per cubic metre), and the much less dense air (around 1.3 kg per cubic metre at a pressure of 1 atmosphere, at sea level and temperature of 4 degrees Celsius). The viscosity of the two fluids is very different too.

The Navier-Stokes equations are over 150 years old, but even today a legion of physicists, engineers and mathematicians keep investigating their qualitative, analytical and quantitative aspects. To the day, the solutions' stability, uniqueness, and direct numerical approximation are difficult and fascinating fields of investigation. In particular, the larger the *Reynolds number*, a parameter equal to the product of the boat's speed times its length, times the inverse of the fluid viscosity, the more complex the numerical approximation will be. It is easy to imagine, then, that modelling the motion of an America's Cup sailing craft, whose Reynolds number may equal a few million, is a very challenging goal.

As we have said already, we do not have an explicit formula for the exact solution of the equations, so we have to resort to their numerical approximation. To that end we draw over the boat's surface a grid (or mesh) made of hundreds of thousands of small triangles (see Fig. 5.3, showing a portion of the submerged part). The process generates a lattice of millions of tetrahedra (called *elements*) in the computational domain Ω.

This discretisation process—skipping all intermediate passages—leads to a system of nonlinear algebraic equations, whose dimension is usually proportional to the number of elements. By the way, in a turbulent regime the elements should, in theory, be small enough to capture the energy exchange mechanisms. These happen inside increasingly smaller vortices, and when the latter become infinitesimal the energy within is dissipated as heat. This *energy*

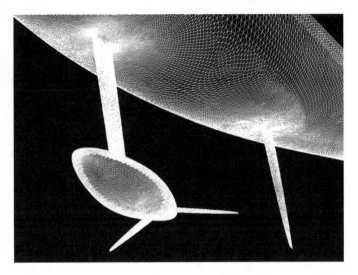

Fig. 5.3 Detail of the surface grid on the submerged part of the vessel

cascade derives its name from the famous Russian scientist Andrej Kolmogorov.

The flow around a sailboat of America's Cup class displays during a race a turbulent behaviour in proximity of most of the wet surface. Turbulent flows are characterised by a non-stationary behaviour, and exhibit coherent (recognisable) vortex structures that interact with one another, exchange energy and fluctuate in time and space. Under these conditions it is unthinkable to simulate the Navier-Stokes equations *directly*, that is, by an approximation involving elements so small that allow to capture all the significant coherent structures. We would need far too many triangles and tetrahedra, so many that no existing computer would be able to manage the problem. Hence one relies on so-called *turbulence models*, obtained by taking suitable averages in the Navier-Stokes equations.

This is most certainly not the end of the story. We now must account for the deformation of the sails, which are elastic. The corresponding equation translates the equilibrium condition for the forces that act on the sails, which are three- or two-dimensional structures (depending on whether or not we take sail thickness into account).

At last, we must write the equations of rigid body dynamics applied to the vessel. For this the diagrams of forces and momenta in Fig. 5.4 will be useful.

So here is our problem, whose solution will faithfully reconstruct the conditions of the regatta: fluid velocity and pressure in each tiny element (of water and air), displacement of every micro-portion of sail, drag forces (including

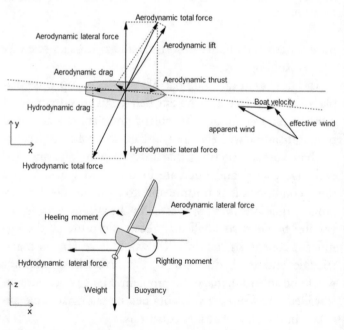

Fig. 5.4 Forces and momenta acting on the boat

the important forces caused by turbulence) acting on every microportion of hull, keel, bulb and winglets [1, 2].

Navier-Stokes equations:

$$\frac{\partial}{\partial t}\left(\overbrace{\rho}\ \underbrace{\vec{v}}\right) + \vec{\nabla}\cdot\left(\rho\vec{v}\otimes\vec{v}\right) - \vec{\nabla}\cdot\overleftrightarrow{\tau}\left(\vec{v}, \underbrace{p}\right) = \rho\,\overrightarrow{g}$$

fluid density — Cauchy stress tensor — gravitational acceleration

fluid velocity — fluid pressure

$$\frac{\partial\rho}{\partial t} + \overrightarrow{\vec{\nabla}}\cdot\left(\rho\vec{v}\right) = 0$$

spatial divergence

Sails equation:

$$\overbrace{\rho_v}\frac{\partial^2\overrightarrow{d}}{\partial t^2} - \vec{\nabla}\cdot\underbrace{\overleftrightarrow{\sigma}_v\left(\overrightarrow{d}\right)} = \overrightarrow{f}_v$$

density of fabric — sail displacement — weight (force)

acceleration term — mechanical stress

Boat's dynamics equation:

$$\underbrace{m}\,\overbrace{\ddot{\vec{X}}}_G = \vec{F}$$

linear acceleration of the yacht's center of mass

mass of yacht

transformation matrix
from fixed to inertial frame   angular velocity

$$\overset{\frown}{\vec{\vec{T}}\,\vec{\vec{I}}\,\vec{\vec{T}}^{-1}}\overset{\rightarrow}{\dot{\Omega}} + \overset{\frown}{\vec{\Omega}} \times \overset{\frown}{\vec{\vec{T}}\,\vec{\vec{I}}\,\vec{\vec{T}}^{-1}}\overrightarrow{\Omega} = \vec{M}_G$$

force due to the
interaction with flow   external force

$$\vec{F} = \overset{\frown}{\vec{F}_{flux}} + m\vec{g} + \overset{\frown}{\vec{F}_{ext}}$$

momentum due to the
interaction with flow

$$\vec{M}_G = \overset{\frown}{\vec{M}_{flux}} + \left(\vec{X}_{ext} - \vec{X}_G\right) \times \vec{F}_{ext}$$

In truth, the Navier-Stokes equations should be rewritten to account for turbulent effects, for instance by splitting the variables into averaged terms plus a correction provided by extra terms that represent the fluctuations. This involves adapting the equation of conservation of momentum, where a viscosity appears that depends non-linearly on the velocity, and also new terms representing the turbulent stresses. To complete the new system it is necessary to introduce two further transport-diffusion equations, one for the turbulent kinetic energy and one for its dissipation rate [1, 2]. At last, let us remark that the Navier-Stokes equations should be written for both air and water, keeping in account the corresponding densities and viscosities. This requires yet another two equations of dynamical and kinematic type at the boundary separating air and water (the free surface), plus an extra equation prescribing the motion of the boundary itself. As one can see, the full mathematical model for the study of an America's Cup sailboat gives the chills to even the best sea-trained mathematicians [3, 4].

5.3   The Numerical Simulations

Once we got a model we were able to address numerical simulations, which mainly regarded three aspects: the analysis of the various configurations of the keel appendices; the behaviour of the free surface around the hull (the wave shape) and its interaction with the appendices; the aerodynamic flow around the sails [5]. The computations provided the design team with an ample assortment of information, which were implemented at different stages of the design cycle. They were even used once the race had started, to suitably adapt the shape of several components (Fig. 5.5).

The keel appendices are a key factor in the success of an America's Cup sailboat. They must guarantee high

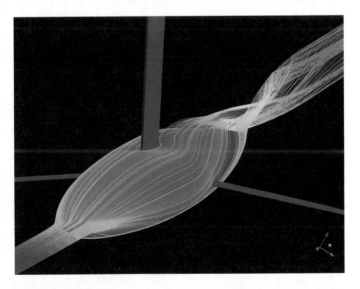

Fig. 5.5   Flow lines around and past the bulb

performances in different regatta conditions (upwind and downwind) and in a wide range of wind conditions, hence of boat velocity.

We considered several design parameters. Regarding the shape of the bulb we analysed various lateral and vertical profiles and many transversal sections, each one having its own plusses and minuses. Elongated bulbs, for instance, allow to reduce the pressure drag, but due to the wider wet surface they undergo a bigger friction.

Winglets were adopted for the first time by Australia II, the 1983 champion. They have been extensively employed by almost all participants to the following editions. Their presence at the bottom of the keel (in analogy to the winglets on aircraft wings) allows to reduce the vortices at those points and decrease a component of the drag known as (lift-)induced drag (Fig. 5.6). Despite winglets have been

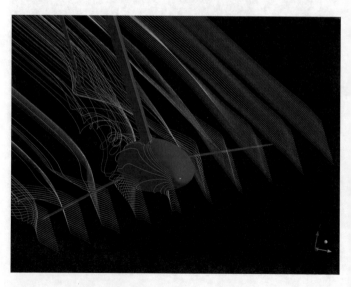

Fig. 5.6 Pressure distribution on the surface of the appendices and flow lines around the winglets

used by every team since, their optimisation with regards to various parameters (longitudinal position, angle of attack, twist and sweep angles and wingplan form) is still an open problem.

In America's Cup monohull boats, wave drag can represent a very significant part (up to 60%) of the total drag. An accurate prediction of this component is therefore decisive during the design phase. To do that numerical methods are required that simulate the dynamics of the free surface separating the air from the water (the wave shape). Using our numerical simulations we examined several winglet shapes, focussing on the bow area.

The aerodynamics of sails is another determining factor. We considered three specific aspects: the estimated forces acting on the sails in downwind leg, the interaction of two competing yachts' sails, the sheltered region created by a windward opponent. Thanks to the analysis of the propulsion force, the lateral force and the pressure distribution, one deduces that the sails work as a combination of a parachute (when the lift is aligned with the direction of thrust) and a vertical wing (with thrust-aligned drag), as was observed by Richards [6].

On downwind leg, the boat sailing to windward has a tactical advantage, since it can control the rival and keep them in the sheltered region, thus significantly reducing wind. We made numerical simulations of the flow around the two boats in downwind leg, and we saw that the flow witnessed by the leeward boat was vastly perturbed by the other vessel. The pressure distributions on the two boats' sails are substantially different (as shown in Figs. 5.7 and 5.8). Information of this kind, extracted from the numerical simulations, is useful during the race as well: it supports the tactical decisions and helps maximise the overbearing on the leeward yacht or curb the negative effects [7, 8].

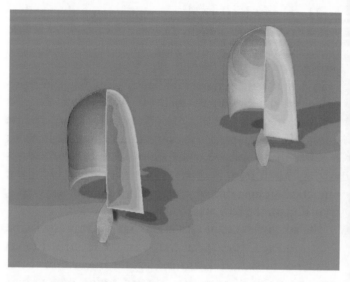

Fig. 5.7 Pressure distribution on the two boats in downwind leg

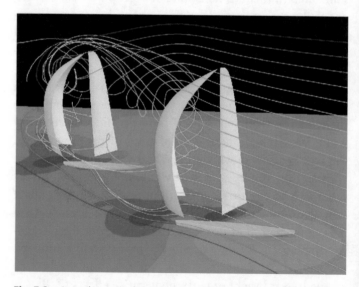

Fig. 5.8 Aerodynamical interaction of two boats sailing downwind

5.4 How Did It End Up?

On 19 January 2003, Alinghi, helmed by Russell Coutts, defeats 4–1 Larry Ellison's *Oracle BMW Racing* US yacht, steered by another New Zealander, Chris Dickinson, and conquers the Louis Vuitton Cup. At EPFL we are flabbergasted: it seems like we are living a dream.

The final race starts on 15 February and the challengers are up against the Black Magic Kiwis. On the 2nd of March, after five successful regattas, Alinghi triumphs: it is the first European team to win the America's Cup. And it is a team from a mountainous, landlocked country!

The 32nd edition was held in Valencia, Spain, by decision of the winning ship owner (called the defender). The challenger is Emirates Team New Zealand (after prevailing 5–0 over the Italian Luna Rossa in the Louis Vuitton Cup final). The decisive race happens between 23 June–9 July 2007, and once again Alinghi wins.

In the 33rd edition, again held in the Valencia waters from the 1st to the 25th of February 2010, Alinghi is defeated by team Oracle's trimaran USA17 steered by James Spithill. This happened after a complex legal battle that gave the Americans a massive advantage from the outset. The racing yachts were significantly different: USA17 had three hulls whereas Alinghi 5 had two; a 68 m mast for the Americans against a "mere" 62 m for the Swiss, a rigid wing as opposed to a mobile sail, the US boat's 17 tons against Alinghi's 11. In a nutshell, it was a technologically uneven race, with an almost foregone outcome.

Alinghi's adventure ends with that third final in seven years, and so does my personal venture in the America's Cup. In the ensuing years I was contacted by other teams, but I preferred to wrap it up with the Swiss experience. My mathematical adventures in high-level sports did not end with sailing, though. Alinghi was without a doubt an important stepping stone, that later on allowed me to engage—mathematically speaking!—in various sports such as rowing, swimming, volleyball and (of course) football. The general goal is to transfer to many sports contexts the knowledge of mathematical modelling, *big data* science, artificial intelligence and *machine learning*. The aim is to improve athletes' individual performances and the strategies and tactics of team sports: an exciting way to use mathematics at the highest levels.

References

1. Parolini N., Quarteroni A. (2005), Mathematical Models and Simulation for the America's Cup, Computer Methods in Applied Mechanics and Engineering, 194, pp. 1001-1026.
2. Parolini N., Quarteroni A. (2004), Simulazione numerica per la Coppa America di vela, Bollettino U.M.I., Serie VIII, 7A, pp. 1-15.
3. Mohammadi P., Pironneau O. (1994), Analysis of the K-Epsilon Turbulence Model, Masson, Paris.
4. Cowles G., Parolini N., Sawley M. (2003), Numerical Simulation using RANS-based Tools for America's Cup Design, Proceedings of the 16th Chesapeake Sailing Yacht Symposium, Annapolis, MD.
5. Quarteroni A. (2009), Mathematical Models in Science and Engineering, Notices of the AMS, 56 (1), pp. 10-19.
6. Richards P.J., Jonhson A., Stanton S. (2001), America's Cup Downwind Sails–Vertical Wings or Horizontal Parachutes?, Journal of Wind Engineering and Industrial Aerodynamics, 89, pp. 1565-1577.
7. Quarteroni A., Sala M., Sawley M.L., Parolini N., Cowles G. W. (2003), Mathematical Modelling and Visualisation of Complex Three-dimensional Flows, in Hege H.C., Polthier K. (Eds.), Visualisation and Mathematics III, Springer, Heidelberg-Berlin.
8. Parolini N., Quarteroni A. (2004), Numerical Simulation for Yacht Design, Proceedings of the 6th Conference on Informatics and Mathematics, Athens, hercma 2003 (E.A. Lipitakis Ed.), 1, pp. 38-44.

6

Flying on Sun Power

Abstract Technology and sustainability: this is the challenge of Solar Impulse, an experimental solar-powered aircraft designed to circumnavigate the globe. Mathematical techniques in multi-objective optimisation have allowed to accommodate the multiple design needs arising from different areas, like materials science, propulsion and aerodynamics.

The dream of flying is as old as the world: just think of Leonardo da Vinci's magnificent yet unachievable machines. More than a century after the Wright brothers' first flight on the dunes of Kitty Hawk, North Carolina, on 17 December 1903, and following the enormous expansion of trade routes across the world, a new era in the history of aviation may be beginning: the challenge of lighter and cleaner aircrafts. On 4 March 2005 Steve Fossett, a man used to great records, landed the *Virgin Atlantic GlobalFlyer*

© The Author(s), under exclusive license to Springer Nature Switzerland AG 2022
A. Quarteroni, *Modeling Reality with Mathematics*,
https://doi.org/10.1007/978-3-030-96162-6_6

in Salina, Kansas, after the first non-stop solo flight around the globe. He flew 67 hours, 2 minutes and 38 seconds on a single turbofan engine [1]. In parallel NASA inaugurated in 1999 the *Helios Prototype* programme, aimed at building a solar-powered, ultra-light experimental aircraft. In 2001 the prototype unofficially broke the world record by reaching the altitude of 29,524 m. The enterprise did not have a happy ending though: on 26 June 2003 the aircraft crashed into the Pacific ocean due to severe instability issues.

The baton was picked up by Bertrand Piccard, who in 2003 launched the Solar Impulse project, a solar-powered aircraft for circumnavigating the earth without stopover. The challenge is blending mankind's dream of adventure and discovery with the respect for the environment, and primarily promote the idea that technology can evolve with clear objectives for sustainable development (Fig. 6.1).

The École Polytechnique Fédérale de Lausanne (EPFL) acted as scientific consultant during the design phase of the

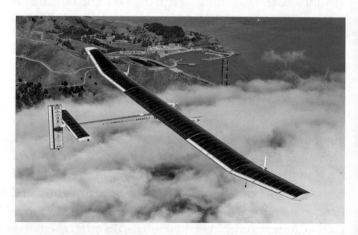

Fig. 6.1 Solar Impulse, a project for the first solar-powered circumnavigation of the globe. Photo: Frederic Legrand—COMEO/Shutterstock

Solar Impulse prototype, by providing human and scientific resources from over ten fields of knowledge, including ultralight materials, energy storage and transformation and new man-machine interface paradigms [2].

My CMCS team came up with the mathematical model in the earliest phase of conceptual design, using techniques called *multi-objective optimisation*. These techniques are essential to find solutions that harmonise design requirements stemming from a number of different contexts (here, materials science, propulsion and aerodynamics), which precisely for their diversity might be conflicting. But before we talk about models let us review some history.

6.1 The Piccards, a Family of Explorers

The Piccards, from Auguste to his grandson Bertrand, passing through Jacques (son of Auguste), are intrepid by family tradition. Auguste Piccard, born in 1884 in Basel, was professor of physics at ETH, the Federal Institute of Technology in Zurich (where Einstein studied and taught) and then at Brussels University. A friend of Albert Einstein and Marie Curie, he contributed to modern aviation and space exploration, inventing the pressurised gondola and the stratospheric balloon. He explored the stratosphere in 1931 and 1932, reaching an altitude of 15,781 and 16,201 m respectively, in order to study cosmic rays. On those occasions he was the first man to observe the curvature of the Earth with his own eyes. He applied the same principle of stratospheric ballooning to the exploration of the oceans' depths, and built a revolutionary submarine called *Bathyscaphe*. Along with his son Jacques, he dove in the bathyscaphe to the depth of 3150 m, thus becoming the *man of the two extremes*: no one before him had flown to such an altitude and explored the ocean abyss.

Jacques Piccard, born in Brussels in 1922, started out reading economics. Because of his contacts in the world of finance he was able to gather the money to fund his father's second bathyscaphe (called *Trieste*). He then abandoned his career and started working with Auguste on the submarine's construction. Together with his father he broke several records, among which the deepest location ever reached: the bottom of the Mariana Trench, at a depth of 10,196 m. After his father's death he carried out the family tradition by constructing four mesoscaphes (submarines for medium depths) including the famous *Auguste Piccard*, the world's first passenger submarine. (During Lausanne's 1964 national exhibition 33,000 tourists explored the depths of Lake Geneva in the *Auguste*.) Among other vehicles we mention the *Ben Franklin*, with which Jacques studied the Gulf current covering 3000 km in one month in 1969, and the *F.-A. Forel*, a easily transportable submersible in which he went on more than 2000 scientific and didactical missions in European lakes and in the Mediterranean.

Bertrand Piccard was born in Lausanne in 1958. Since an early age he was interested in studying the human behaviour in extreme conditions. He was one of the pioneers of hang gliding and micro-light flying in the 1970s, and became European hang-glider aerobatics champion in 1985. After switching to ballooning, in 1992 he won with Wim Verstraeten the first transatlantic balloon race (the Chrysler Challenge). He then launched the Breitling Orbiter project (Fig. 6.2), a vehicle designed for flying non-stop around the globe, and piloted all three successive attempts (alas, all failed). In 1999, along with the British aviator Brian Jones, Piccard completed the first balloon flight around the globe, which was also the longest flight ever made for distance and

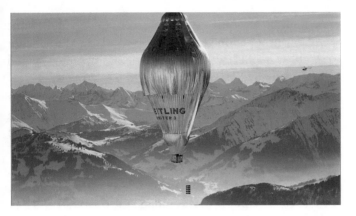

Fig. 6.2 The Breitling Orbiter 3. Foto: Cedric Favero / VWPics / Alamy Foto Stock

duration. They took off in Switzerland and landed in Egypt after 19 days and 21 hours, from 1 to 20 March 1999 [3]. In 2003, as mentioned, he embarked on the Solar Impulse enterprise, which besides an adventure is also a project bearing important technological and social commitments.

6.2 Ending the Fossil-Fuel Era

To the day the primary energy source and the bedrock of the global economy is oil. Its derivatives are everywhere: fuel for cars, aeroplanes and heating systems, asphalt for roads, plastic components and so on. But this resource is finite. It is estimated that the planet's reserves amount to 3000 billion barrels. At the start of this millennium 1000 have been already depleted, 1000 have been discovered and another 1000 are still to be found (this estimate has the advantage of being easy: one third, one third, one third).

According to some studies, in certain regions of the world oil production has already peaked (in the US, for example, it might have happened in November 2017), and is now declining. Some predict that the reserves will be exhausted within 50 years. These studies are based on the assumption that oil consumption has a constant growth in time, so that a small fluctuation in the global demand would suffice to change these numbers.

Perhaps the most plausible scenario is different, though, and we will not reach the point of exhausting resources completely. According to this model, the reserves' depletion will make the price of oil increase until it will be no longer profitable to extract it. Another factor that will curb the use of oil derivatives is the increase of greenhouse gases in the atmosphere. Greenhouse gases, in particular water vapour (H_2O), ozone (O_3) and carbon dioxide (CO_2), usually considered the main culprits of global warming, are mostly produced when burning fossil fuels. According to NASA's *Earth Observatory*, if we take into account the plausible scenarios of fossil energy consumption the average temperature on Earth may increase by 2–6 °C by the end of the twenty-first century. Part of this warming will happen anyway, even if we reduce greenhouse gas emissions, because of the inertial effect due to the adjustment of system Earth to environmental changes that have already occurred [4]. The global climate will change radically: the polar caps will melt, sea levels will rise, tropical storms will become more severe, ecosystems will be destroyed. Given the complexity and interdependence of the phenomena we are considering, the degree of reliability of these analyses is clearly not the highest.

One other thing is certain: at the end of this century our society will be completely different from the one we know now. We are all aware we must decide whether to maintain the current dynamics and bear the brunt (which might be dramatic), or try to steer course with a gradual transition to energy forms that are alternative to fossil fuels. For this to happen it is necessary to promote the idea of *sustainable growth*, that is, meeting the needs of the present without compromising the chances of future generations of meeting theirs. There is no doubt science will have to play a crucial role in this transition phase.

6.3   The Solar Impulse Mission: The Challenges

The *Solar Impulse* project was born, among other things, precisely to promote sustainable growth. It uses renewable energy, stimulates the susceptibility to environmental issues and strengthens the idea that technology can help create a novel model of growth. The project's ultimate objective was to fly around the globe an aircraft powered by green energy only (in particular, solar energy) and free of polluting emissions. Mission accomplished: the aircraft left Abu Dhabi on 9 March 2015 headed eastbound, and returned there on 26 July 2016, more than 16 months later (it had to make a long stop-over to repair the significant battery damage caused by heat on the longest stretch, from Japan to Hawaii, in July 2015).

The design of an aircraft of this kind requires that we address several technological challenges. The main one is to optimise energy harvesting and consumption. Considering atmospheric absorption and cloud reflection, the sunlight power reaching the Earth is about 1020 kW/m^2 (at sea level). That is quite a number: the solar radiation hitting the entire surface of the Earth *every* minute exceeds the annual energy consumption of the whole planet. The Sun could therefore meet our energy demand, if only we were able to exploit it properly. On the other hand it is clear that the Sun is not a regular source of energy: it is obviously not available in areas under the cover of darkness. So we must find a way to store energy for later use, and one of the key aspects of the project was exactly to maximise solar energy accumulation. Wide wings were chosen to accommodate large photovoltaic cells and high-capacity power batteries. During the cruise of *Solar Impulse*, the harvested energy can be handled in two ways: it is stored in the batteries to increase the energy reserve for the night, or it gets used immediately to power the electric engines.

Choosing a large wingspan allows to maximise solar energy harvest in daylight, but it reflects negatively on the structural aspects, since the aircraft becomes heavier and hence it uses up more energy. To remedy the problem it then becomes essential to involve last-generation, ultralight composite materials.

The aircraft is also subjected to big temperature variations during the mission, at different times of day and different altitudes. The temperature difference between the upper and lower wing surface can reach 60 °C at peak exposition to sunlight. Moreover, the batteries become less efficient when it is too cold (typically, below 0 °C). So it is necessary to isolate the batteries inside the wings and guarantee the materials do not undergo thermal shocks that might compromise functionality.

A further (and certainly fundamental) challenge regards the pilot's safety. In daylight, *Solar Impulse* reaches altitudes beyond 10,000 m, where the temperature goes below -50 °C and the air is extremely rarefied. So one needs an efficient thermal insulation and a suitable pressurisation system. Moreover, an automatic steering system must be designed to avoid an excessive burden on the pilot over long hauls.

Many challenges and demands, at times contrasting: all of which has made the design of the solar aircraft a true technological bet. Therefore every design choice was carefully examined, because it has a potentially great impact on the general behaviour of the aircraft.

6.4 Mathematics Comes into Play

To design *Solar Impulse* it became necessary to literally rethink the concept of aircraft. Its configuration could not be extrapolated from existent ones or from standard design strategies. One had to develop aerodynamical models anew, for the structural behaviour's analysis, the handling of energy and propulsion, and for integrating these under a global optimisation framework.

In a case like this, it is not possible to keep the involved fields separated and try to optimise the single components independently, because the specific choices in one aspect of the project could strongly affect the system's behaviour in other contexts. The only possible approach is then an integrated optimisation strategy, that accounts for the different components and their interactions (we will see some details in the following section).

The *Solar Impulse* project is based on mathematical models of high complexity, which translate into algorithms with great computational costs. Hence it becomes necessary to come up with simplified models. Luckily, aerodynamics is one typical field where it is possible to define a *hierarchy of models*, each with different levels of completeness, precision and computational complexity, that can be integrated efficiently.

Let us consider for instance how to address the problem of designing the profiles of wings and stabilisers, whose aim is to reduce air drag and optimise the aircraft's efficiency and stability. For this we shall use a so-called *potential-flow model* [5], which simplifies reality in one precise respect: it is founded on the assumption that the flow is irrotational (also known as curl-free), meaning there are no vortices. In this way the model is very efficient computationally (calculations take little time). A potential-flow model is used to study the wing's aerodynamical behaviour, that is, to predict air drag, cruising speed and lift (which, being perpendicular to the aircraft's direction of motion, is in practice the component of the force supporting the aircraft). It is also employed to estimate how the air behaves along the wing profile (whether the flow is laminar or turbulent). In order to simulate the 3D flow's behaviour around the aircraft, instead, a *hierarchically higher* model is necessary: the latter is more complete, and is based on the solution to the Navier-Stokes equations [6] we met in the previous chapters.

The passage from the physical model to the computational one is facilitated by programs such as CAD (*Computer Aided Design*), that allow to represent the entire aircraft using a collection of geometrical shapes and define several computational domains. The flow-governing equations, as we have seen elsewhere, must be discretised. To do that we subdivide the three-dimensional domain into a computational grid (or mesh) made of elementary cells, shaped as small pyramids (tetrahedra) or cubes (hexahedra), and we impose that the equations hold locally on each element of the grid.

In order for the simulation to be realistic, the mesh must not be uniform, but should be refined suitably in the areas with *steep gradients*, that is, where the variables describing the solutions (especially velocity, pressure and air

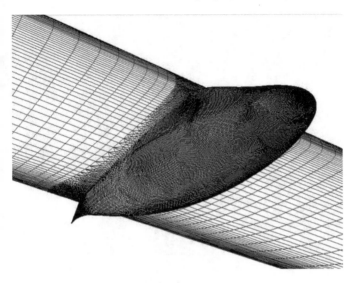

Fig. 6.3 Example of computational mesh

temperature) change suddenly. See Fig. 6.3 for an example. This may lead to a very large number of elements (in the order of millions, or tens of millions for the finest grids) and to algebraic problems of prohibitive dimension, which can be solved only by resorting to algorithms implemented on large parallel-computer architectures.

The results of these numerical simulations are essential to understand in detail how the air flow behaves around the aircraft, and how, in particular, to capture the effects on the overall performance of phenomena such as vortex shedding or the presence of areas of air recirculation.

Figure 6.4 shows two examples of 3D simulations: in the top picture we have the typical vortex at the wing tip, highlighted by the streamlines. Below we see the distribution of pressure values on the wing surface and the engine gondola.

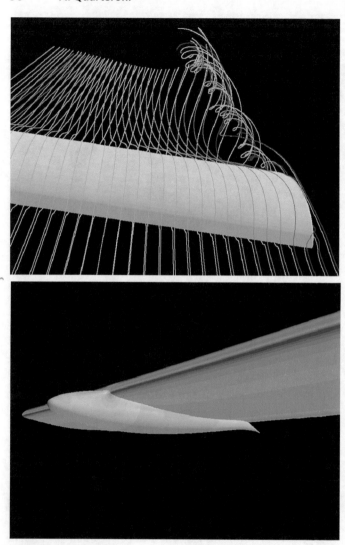

Fig. 6.4 Two examples of 3D airflow simulations around the aircraft

6.5 Multidisciplinary Optimisation

In a complex project like *Solar Impulse* suitable trade-offs must be found to satisfy the needs, at times conflicting, of each component. Consider for example the simple question "how many batteries should be fitted onboard?". As regards the propulsion, the answer is "as many as possible", since the electric energy produced by the photovoltaic cells is the only source available, so we would want to store as much of it as possible. On the other hand batteries are heavy, and too many might compromise the mission, for a number of reasons. First, a bigger weight requires more energy to take the aircraft higher, or just to support it at a constant altitude. Second, batteries must be kept at a temperature as uniform as possible to work properly; increasing their number would require more energy to heat them (it is cold up there). Third, a bigger load would require a more robust structure and hence a further increase of the overall weight of the aircraft. So it is clear that calculating the ideal number of batteries is not easy: we must optimise it and keep many constraints in account at the same time.

Problems of this sort can be tackled using a multidisciplinary optimisation approach. The latter, also known as *multi-objective optimization*, allows to integrate the models used in several fields (here, structural mechanics, aerodynamics, propulsion, thermal analysis). This situation shows up in countless other contexts, say automotive design, where one would like to maximise the performance of a new car and at the same time minimise the consumption and maximise comfort (by reducing noise and vibrations).

The *objective functions* are the quantities to be optimised (either maximised or minimised). The problems typically involve several objective functions. It is easy to imagine that there is no single solution optimising all objective functions, in general. There exist, though, many solutions (theoretically, infinitely many) that represent acceptable trade-offs. Objective functions are called *Pareto optimal*, or *nondominated*, provided they satisfy the following property: none can be improved without degrading some of the others.

We can express the above property more precisely in mathematical terms. Suppose our multi-objective optimisation problem consists in finding a vector x of dimension $n \geq 2$ that minimises the objective functions $f_1(x)$, $f_2(x)$, ..., $f_n(x)$. (Note that there is no loss in generality by assuming we must minimise everything: if one objective function had to be maximised, it would be enough to flip its sign and then minimise. This is a standard trick of mathematicians.)

The *design parameters* are numerical values describing an acceptable configuration. They may be quantities that vary continuously (the wing span, the inclination of the wing profile to the airflow), or in a discrete fashion (number of solar cells, of batteries etc.).

As we said, in general there are no vectors x minimising all objective functions *simultaneously*. So one looks for trade-off solutions, called *Pareto optimal solutions*. Let us start with a definition. We say a solution x_1(Pareto) dominates another solution x_2 if $f_i(x_1)$ is less than or equal to $f_i(x_2)$ for all indices $i = 1,...,n$, and if for at least one index j, $f_j(x_1)$ is strictly smaller than $f_j(x_2)$. A solution is then Pareto optimal whenever there is no solution dominating it. The collection of optimal solutions is the so-called *Pareto front*.

Figure 6.5 shows a simple example with $n = 2$. The points A and B, on the Pareto front, represent optimal solutions. The point C and all lighter-coloured squares are non-optimal solutions.

As we observed, multi-objective optimisation is a process that allows to select the best configuration in high-complexity systems, by keeping into account the

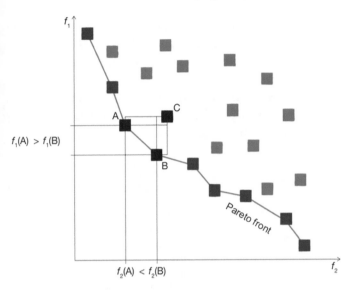

Fig. 6.5 Two Pareto optimal solutions A and B

interactions among the project's many aspects. In other words, it aims to find a mathematical answer to the following key question: how does one decide what to change in a configuration, and when to change it, if every design parameter affects everything else?

6.6 An Example of Multi-objective Optimisation

Now let us take a look at a concrete example. The question is: what is the maximum weight allowed for the structure of *Solar Impulse* if we want to fly at night above a pre-established altitude? Answering the question helps designers determine, say, the type of composite material for the wing structure. It is a real and concrete problem, which we addressed in the EPFL labs by considering the aircraft's structural, aerodynamical and electric characteristics. Objective functions, design variables and constraints are defined in Table 6.1.

The realisable configurations obtained from the model are shown in Fig. 6.6. We examined 20,000 configurations and saw that four thousand satisfied the constraints. The

Table 6.1 Objective functions, design parameters and constraints to find the maximum weight allowed

Objective functions
  Maximisation of minimal nocturnal altitude
  Maximisation of structure's weight
Design parameters
  Wingspan = 80 m
  Wing surface = 230 sq. m
  Battery weight = 450 kg
  Structure's weight = 800–1000 kg
Constraints
  Minimal nocturnal altitude > 3000 m

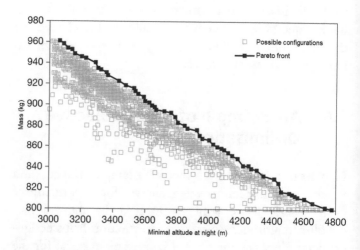

Fig. 6.6 The problem's Pareto front

rightmost boundary of the cluster of points defines the problem's Pareto front.

As we said, selecting configurations on the Pareto front corresponds to fixing a weight (or a coefficient) for each one of the objective functions considered. In mathematical terms, it means finding the coefficients $w_1,...,w_n$ that optimise the function $w_1f_1+...+w_nf_n$. In this case the curve shows the influence of the structure's weight on the minimum altitude reached at night. We discover that, for example, above 1000 kg the constraints are never satisfied, and that if we decided, for safety reasons, to fly above 4000 m at night, the maximum structural weight allowed would be 860 kg. The flight profiles (in terms of altitude and speed) corresponding to the two ends of the curve are shown in Figs. 6.7

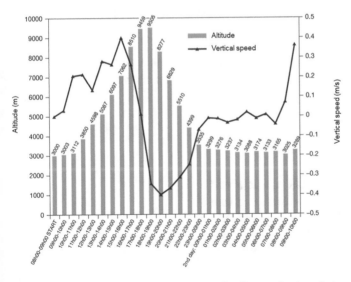

Fig. 6.7 Flight profile corresponding to the first endpoint of the Pareto front

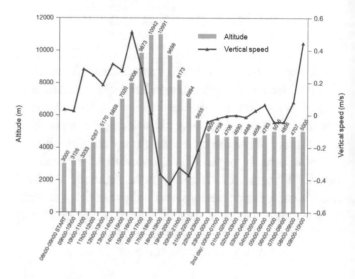

Fig. 6.8 Flight profile corresponding to the second endpoint of the Pareto front

and 6.8. This computation is an example of how multi-objective optimisation can be employed to support design choices.

References

1. www.stevefossett.com *
2. www.solarimpulse.com *
3. www.bertrandpiccard.com *
4. earthobservatory.nasa.gov/features/GlobalWarming *
5. Drela M. (1989), Xfoil: An Analysis and Design System for Low Reynolds Number Airfoils, Lecture Notes in Engineering 54, Springer, New York.
6. Peyret R. (a cura di) (1996), Handbook of Computational Fluid Mechanics, Academic Press, London.

7

The Taste for Mathematics

Abstract Mathematics is useful to model the consistency of chocolate as its temperature varies, to simulate new production chains and to optimise the packaging, storage and transport of food products. This also includes the optimisation of the nutritional content of food in view of maximising flavour perception.

The appreciation of a good meal, the art of cooking, food science, the technology of food preparation: various facets of one of the basic needs of the human being, namely, finding a source of enough energy to make the body function on a daily basis. Food processing has passed from being artisanal to becoming an important industry that sees the growing involvement of multinationals operating on a global scale. Although it may seem surprising, in recent years the food industry has formed an increasingly tighter

© The Author(s), under exclusive license to Springer Nature Switzerland AG 2022
A. Quarteroni, *Modeling Reality with Mathematics*,
https://doi.org/10.1007/978-3-030-96162-6_7

bond with mathematics, which is often (wrongly) seen as the science most detached from the primary needs of human beings.

7.1   Food Preparation

The food industry has been, for a while now, a testing ground for the application of mathematical models. Before we go to concrete examples, let us use a scheme to summarise the typical path of a product in the food supply chain. Even if simplistic, it will give us an idea of the complexity of the process. A specific product may be thought of as the creation of a team of specialised researchers, who work to devise better food for nutritional value, flavour, aspect and attractiveness to consumers. Apart from its intrinsic characteristics, it is useful to study the way this product will be prepared, its packaging, the conservation of its properties along the route that includes distribution, sale and arrival to the end consumer's home. Figure 7.1 shows three steps, where we have highlighted the contributions mathematics can offer.

Even after sale and consumption, the product can be studied. For instance, we can examine how much the consumer liked it and which effects it has on health (good or bad). In these circumstances, too, mathematics can reveal very useful. In the following sections we will see some examples.

7.2   Mathematics and the Brain

What links the perception of taste through the taste buds to the corresponding sensation elaborated by the brain? It is a process we pay no attention to, that repeats daily. Yet it is

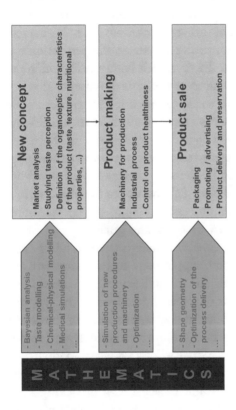

Fig. 7.1 When a food product encounters mathematics

extraordinarily complex, for it involves a particularly difficult organ to model, the brain. The *Brain and Mind Institute* at EPFL [1] aims to create models capable of emulating the brain activity, using a supercomputer that performs more than 300,000 billion operations per second. That is an incredible speed, necessary to reproduce the actions and interactions of hundreds of thousands of nerve cells at a time. One aspect of this very ambitious study is directed at simulating the processes that govern the perception and evaluation of taste. These models compute the brain's energy requirements and try to optimise the composition of nutrients in food, with particular attention for two consumer groups in critical phases of life: small children and elderly people.

It is known that the first assessment of a food happens through the eyes, and that our choices concerning food are often guided by the appearance of what stands in front of us. The *Blue Brain* [2] project has the objective of analysing the cognitive processes of sight, beside the more primary processes relative to taste and smell.

Thanks to *Blue Brain* neuroscientists will be able to conduct computer experiments to test diagnostic and therapeutical tools for neurodegenerative diseases. Numerical models allow to make simulations of the biophysical processes happening at the various levels of the cerebral architecture, thus integrating the morphological and structural data of a single brain with a universal mathematical model based on a representation of the biochemical and electric activity at the cellular level. Today, modelling a single nerve cell requires we solve a system of 20,000 ordinary differential equations, roughly. This number mushrooms to more than 100 billion if we want to model the entire brain activity. A goal that is still very far away.

7.3   The "Formula of Flavour"

Taste is the most immediate and important sense presiding over our relationship with food. Therefore managing flavour is the primary task, and the most complex one, in the industrial design of food. A product's flavour is created by mixing several ingredients, among which there may be preservants, colour additives or artificial aromas, which clearly do not appear in the homemade version of the same recipe. Understanding how a certain quantity of a certain substance will affect the final taste of a product is almost never an easy process. For that reason some companies rely on mathematics to gain more insight on the matter, preferably in a deterministic, and hence reproducible, way. Researchers at Glasgow University, for instance, have developed the *formula of flavour* for blackcurrant drinks, which provides the expected result when using the basic ingredients [3]. The starting point is based on neural networks, to which we shall return in the next chapter, and allows to calculate the intensity of blackcurrant flavour as one tweaks the relative ingredients' quantities. It also takes into account variables such as the berries' geographical provenance and the harvest period. Another mathematical model has been developed, again at the University of Glasgow, to study the relationship between the sweet flavour of lager and the presence of volatile substances other than sugar in the mix (in this case, too, with the help of neural networks) [4].

The success of an industrially processed food is not only a matter of flavour, though. Also texture plays an important role in steering consumer choices. To this end researchers at Birmingham University studied heat conduction in chocolate to predict the product's consistency in function of its temperature [5]. The hardening process of chocolate has several critical components, and depends not only on the initial and final temperatures, but also on the cooling time and on the end product's desired shape. Everything starts with the heat equation [6], which predicts how temperature will propagate in the chocolate. In particular, it is a good idea to control the cooling strategy to guarantee that the transition from the liquid phase to the solid phase is as efficient as possible.

The physics of heat transfer also governs a process particularly dear to Italians: the cooking of pasta, an (almost) daily action for many of us.

The necessary chemical and physical transformations (starch gelatinisation, denaturation, and coagulation of gluten, essentially) happen only if the water reaches a certain temperature. Contrary to the common belief, this is not 100 degrees Celsius, the boiling point; it suffices, in fact, to maintain the liquid at 80–85 degrees. The ideal cooking time depends on a number of factors, not least our personal taste. But it is possible to obtain a simple formula [7], different for each type of pasta. For spaghetti we have

$$t = ar^2 + b$$

where a is a coefficient that depends on the manufacturing, r is the spaghetti radius and b is another coefficient reflecting the desired cooking level (small for *al dente* pasta, large if we want it well cooked). The formula for *bucatini*, instead, accounts for the hollow shape. In this case

$$t = \frac{a(D-d)^2}{2} + b$$

where D and d are the outer and inner diameters respectively.

7.4 Optimising the Industrial Production of Food

Industrial food production consists, concretely, in a series of chemical and physical transformations of the basic ingredients. Each one of its phases can therefore be examined with the aid of mathematics. Let us see some examples.

The Mechanical Engineering Department at University of Padua has analysed the molecular viscosity of dough inside an industrial mixer, and the study's results have prompted the modification of the machine to improve its performance. The dough for fresh pasta, like many other foods, behaves like a *non-Newtonian fluid*. This is a fluid whose viscosity is not constant (as opposed to the classical case of a *Newtonian* fluid, like air, or water) but depends on its velocity. Hence the classical behavioural models of viscid fluids inside machines such as mixers should be substituted by new models, which account for this feature and treat viscosity as a variable rather than as a constant. Non-Newtonian fluids, by the way, have become familiar to the general public in the last few years because they lend themselves well to spectacular demonstrations. Most of us have come across videos on the internet of researchers *walking on water*, that is, walking without sinking over a pool filled with a milky-looking liquid. Usually that liquid is a mixture of water and corn or potato starch. The stunt is possible because the force applied by the foot pressing onto the surface makes the fluid behave like a solid rather than a liquid. A weaker force, like that of a spoon in a liquid, does not cause any apparent change in state [8].

The Department of Mathematics at University of Florence, instead, concerned itself with coffee. A research group studied the way in which pressurised water filters through the coffee powder, to establish which conditions lead to the formation of lumps. This phenomenon alters the transfer of the aroma from the coffee powder to the water, and hence it changes the taste of the beverage [9]. While Italian universities study pasta and coffee (no surprise there), in California, as one might imagine, the focus is on hamburgers and on finding out the best way to cook them to optimise flavour, digestibility and food safety. Cooking a hamburger is a less trivial task than we might expect. One must determine precisely the temperature and cooking time, so to eliminate the possible pathogens present in the meat without altering too much its nutritional value and (most of all) the mouth-watering taste. The *Food and Drug Administration* (the American agency responsible for the safety of food and drugs) has issued precise regulations regarding the minimum temperature and cooking time of hamburgers prepared by the food industry or restaurants. At the root of it all lies a physics problem: how can one make the heat propagate inside the meat so that each part reaches the minimum required temperature? It is easy to imagine that the solution depends in an essential way on the hamburger's shape and thickness. The corresponding mathematical model is provided by the following equation, which does not look very complicated but in truth requires non-trivial solution techniques:

$$\frac{\partial H}{\partial t} = \frac{\partial}{\partial z}\left(k \frac{\partial T}{\partial z} \right) + \frac{1}{r}\frac{\partial}{\partial r}\left(rk \frac{\partial T}{\partial r} \right).$$

Here H is the enthalpy (the sum of the internal energy and the product of the pressure p by the volume V), k is the thermal conductivity inside the meat (in turn depending on the enthalpy), t is time, T the temperature, r the radial coordinate (going from the centre to the periphery) and z the vertical coordinate (measuring thickness).

The model must be completed with several other equations, expressing the outward heat flow from the crust, and suitable transfer conditions between the hamburger's frozen and defrosted parts (a complex free-boundary mathematical problem!). According to this model, a standard double grill heated at 200 degrees Celsius needs about 120 seconds to make the centre of a 1.1 cm thick hamburger reach 75 degrees, exactly matching the experimental evidence! [10].

In the last few years other American teams have studied the thermal behaviour of several liquids (milk, apple juice, tomato sauce etc.) when they are hit by a microwave beam, a very common procedure in the food industry [11]. To tackle that problem it is necessary to solve Maxwell's equations, which lie at the heart of every electromagnetic phenomenon. Important domestic-appliance companies study how to optimise irradiation so that a specific food (say, chicken) is cooked in the most uniform possible way depending on its shape and weight.

7.5 Mathematical Packaging

A freshly produced food still has a long way to go before it reaches our dinner table: it must be packaged, distributed to sellers and preserved appropriately. All jobs that mathematics can make more efficient. Let us take packaging. It is necessary to optimise the shape of the packaging and its material to make it robust but light, and able to prevent external contamination. The researchers at Technische Universiteit Eindhoven in the Netherlands are specialised in, thanks to modelling, designing glass bottles [12]. This is another common object that, even if not manifestly, involves advanced technological solutions. Mathematics contributes to the optimisation of shape, weight and rigidity, and helps maximise storage and transport. Ideal bottles, in fact, must be piled up and packaged so to minimise the waste of space. Clearly, one must consider the usability constraints: producing cubical bottles, for instance, would solve the stacking problem mathematically, but certainly not the ease of use.

A research group in Amsterdam, once again in the Netherlands, has applied mathematics to the study of preserving vegetables in modified atmosphere, with the aim of prolonging shelf life [13]. A significant improvement of food preservation techniques can have important consequences on distribution. Thanks to these studies it is now possible to transport fresh produce by sea instead of air, thus lowering the ensuing overall costs.

In general, the task of finding the best way for food to go from the producer to the consumer may be seen as an application of a classical problem in operations research: the *travelling salesman problem* [14]. This problem is easy to state but difficult to solve. Imagine a salesman has to visit a given number of clients scattered in a region in a non-uniform way, and suppose he know the distances between each client, the network of available routes and the travelling times of each. The salesman will want to minimise the effort, that is, travel the least possible. In the past the experienced salesman would have relied on experience, but today we are able of providing precise mathematical solutions to the problem.

We could give other examples of how mathematics applies to packaging and logistics, but now we are hungry: the food has arrived on the table and we can enjoy it.

7.6 Mathematics and Health

A food continues to be the object of mathematical investigation even after it has been eaten. A product's success should be assessed against consumer satisfaction, sure, but also based on its effects, good or bad, on the health of who eat it.

To make a simple example let us mention a study, done with statistical methods, in which a team at University College London has determined the features of the *perfect* product [15]. If you think that in the US almost 90% of newly launched foods are called back after a while because of low sales, it becomes clear that studies of this kind are a new and powerful tool for the people coming up with new products in an ever more competitive market.

Consumers, on the other hand, might judge a product's nutritional value more important than its commercial success.

Another aspect of food distribution that has worldwide relevance is waste prevention. It is estimated that every year 1.3 billion tons of food go wasted: slightly more than half during production and harvest, the rest during processing, distribution and consumption. At the same time 870 million people go hungry every day. By 2050, when the world population will pass the 9 billion threshold, food production will have to increase 70% to feed the entire planet [16]. For this reason the École Polytechnique Fédérale de Lausanne has created the *Integrative Food and Nutrition Center*: to solve the challenges posed by a sustainable future of food and nutrition. The studies conducted at EPFL range from precision agriculture to more efficient packaging systems and a better handling of waste [17].

Today the relationship between eating and mathematics is very tight, as we have seen. In this chapter we have only scratched the surface with the help of examples showing how modelling is omnipresent in every phase of a food product's life. It is interesting to observe that the mathematics necessary to address the problems described here is very complex. These examples reflect a picture of mathematics that is very different from the (wrong) idea of an abstract science, crystallised in a list of theorems that are totally irrelevant to the lay person. It is a mathematics that can accompany us inside the kitchen, advise us and surprise us in ways we could not have imagined [18].

References

1. www.epfl.ch/schools/sv/bmi/ *
2. bluebrain.epfl.ch *
3. Boccorh R.K., Paterson A. (2002), An Artificial Neural Network Model for Predicting Flavour Intensity in Blackcurrant Concentrates , Food Quality and Preference, 13, pp. 117-128.
4. Techakriengkrai I., Paterson A., Piggot J.R. (2004), Relationships of Sweetness in Lager to Selected Volatile Congeners, Journal Institute Brewing, 110 (4), pp. 360-366.
5. Tewkesbury H., Stapley A.G.F., Fryer P.J. (2000), Modelling Temperature Distributions in Cooling Chocolate Moulds, Chemical Engineering Science, 55, pp. 3123-3132.
6. Quarteroni A. Numerical Models of Differential Problems, 3rd edition, Springer Series MS&A, Vol 16, 2017 (xvii+681p.).
7. Rigamonti A., Varlamov A. (2007), Magico caleidoscopio della fisica, La Goliardica Pavese, Pavia.
8. Owens R.G., Phillips T.N. (2002), Computational Rheology, Imperial College Press, London.
9. Fasano A. (1996), Some Non-Standard One-Dimensional Filtration Problems, The Bulletin of Faculty of Education, Chiba University (iii, Natural Sciences), 44, pp. 5-29
10. Singh R.P. (2000), Moving Boundaries in Food Engineering, Food Technology, 54 (2), pp. 44-53.

11. Zhu J., Kuznetsov A.V., Sandeep K.P. (2007), Mathematical Modelling of Continuous Flow Microwave Heating of Liquids (Effects of Dielectric Properties and Design Parameters), International Journal of Thermal Science, 46, pp. 328-341.

12. Laevsky K., Mattheij R.M.M. (2000), Mathematical Modelling of Some Glass Problems, in Fasano A., Complex Flows in Industrial Processes, Birkhäuser, Basel.

13. Rijgersberg, H., Top J.L. (2003), An Engineering Model of Modified Atmosphere Packaging for Vegetables, 2003 International Conference on Bond Graph Modeling and Simulation, Miami, FL.

14. Applegate D.L., Bixby R.E., Chvátal V., Cook W.J. (2006), The Traveling Salesman Problem: A Computational Study, Princeton University Press, Princeton, NJ.

15. Corney D. (2000), Designing food with Bayesian Belief Networks, Proceedings of ACDM2000 – Adaptive Computing in Design and Manufacture, Plymouth, UK.

16. Report 2013, Food and Agriculture Organization of The United Nations.

17. www.epfl.ch/research/domains/nutrition-center1*

18. Giusti E. (2004), La matematica in cucina, Bollati Boringhieri, Torino.

8

The Future Awaiting Us

Abstract Not just models but also artificial intelligence, machine learning and big data. Thanks to the advancements in scientific knowledge and in the computational power of supercomputers, the mathematical models of the future will be increasingly accurate.

Hopefully I have managed to convince the reader that mathematics, just like many other disciplines, is useful, beautiful and creative, and at the same time contributed to debunk a number of misconceptions.

Myth number one: mathematics is a self-referential discipline, practised by individuals that are often incapable of communicating with the world. In reality we have seen that all cases examined required a strong interaction with professionals from other disciplines, whether doctors, meteorologists, athletes or other. For doing good applied mathematics it is necessary to immerse oneself in the problems, capture

© The Author(s), under exclusive license to Springer Nature
Switzerland AG 2022
A. Quarteroni, *Modeling Reality with Mathematics*,
https://doi.org/10.1007/978-3-030-96162-6_8

their essential features and hold regular conversations with other people. My own personal motto in this respect is: tell me what answer you expect and we mathematicians will try to formulate the mathematically most correct question.

Myth number two: there is a clear-cut distinction between pure and applied mathematics. No. There is only one sort of mathematics that makes sense doing—the good sort, and the deeper we know it the better we will manage to apply it to problem-solving. What is true is that there is a difference between pure and applied *mathematicians*, due to a different attitude *when doing mathematics*. Applied mathematicians put the problem to be solved at the centre of their attention (for they feel the need to give the real world answers) and do not accept simplifying compromises if these undermine the result's significance. Pure mathematicians, instead, are interested in the problem's structure, in unearthing the theoretical properties, thus possibly paving the way to the creation of new theories that may lead far away from the study's original motivation. The latter is curiosity-driven research, as opposed to the former's problem-driven research. But the line separating the two scopes is not clear-cut, and the background knowledge is the same. I myself have often moaned about not knowing enough mathematics: sometimes, certain apparently very abstract areas would have helped me build better models, and therefore find more efficient solutions to real problems.

Myth number three: mathematics can be done only by hand. Nothing could be more wrong. What if we did not have computers? Actually: supercomputers, which perform up to one billion billion operations per second (just like *Frontier* at Oak Ridge National Laboratories in the US, the fastest supercomputer in the world at the time of writing). Almost every problem I have discussed in the book has been solved with supercomputers. In order to translate these machines' potential into a real advantage new algorithms had to be developed, called parallel algorithms. It is because of these novel instruments that we can get the most out of machines made by clusters of several thousands of independent logical units, also known as *cores*. This is but one of many examples where technology and research go hand in hand, one amplifying the other's success.

One aspect I did not mention, that nonetheless deserves a few words, is the difference between deterministic models and stochastic models. Here in fact I have concentrated on the former kind exclusively. A process is called *deterministic* if it produces the same solution each time we feed it the same data. We call it *stochastic*, instead, if it keeps into account that the input data may fluctuate in a more or less casual way, and therefore it provides solutions only within a certain probability margin. Examples of stochastic processes are those describing the behaviour of biological systems of human actions (in social phenomena, financial choices, decisions regarding games and competitions). In certain applied contexts resorting to stochastic models is inevitable. Think about climate: foreseeing the average temperature increase in 30–50 years' time necessarily depends on the human footprint in the coming years, for instance, a variable that can only be represented in probabilistic terms. It goes without saying that solving a non-deterministic model is way more complicated than solving a deterministic model.

About that, nowadays there is a very popular technique among mathematicians, called *uncertainty quantification* (UQ). In practice one starts from a deterministic model and assumes that the data oscillate within a confidence interval (represented, say, by a Gaussian distribution). At this point one computes how the uncertainty of the data reverberates on the solution, and then one determines, retroactively, the acceptable confidence interval. These techniques are for instance used in models of the circulatory system (see chapter four) where a lot of data have an intrinsic degree of uncertainty (think of the lack of accuracy in reconstructing the shape of organs from medical images like CT scans or MRIs). They are also employed when the data cannot be generated: this is the case of quantities such as the myocardium's electric conductivity, which is just impossible to quantify on a living being.

The reader who made it to this point might wonder why I did not speak about subjects like artificial intelligence (AI), *machine learning* or *big data*, which dominate the media so much they have become topics of small talk. I have no bias against them whatsoever. I wanted to talk about models simply because it is an approach to problems somehow *alternative* to that of artificial intelligence. AI is a fascinating and complex subject that would deserve a whole new discussion, but I will try to summarise what I mean.

Let us begin from the definitions: *artificial intelligence* is a computer's ability to emulate the cognitive functions of the human mind, such as learning and problem solving. *Machine learning* is a computer's ability to learn and perform a specific action without prior programming via explicit instructions. Although not new (the first definition of AI goes back at least 60 years), these concepts have had a groundbreaking impact only recently. The crucial leap forward is probably due to *big data*, a term referring to the availability of immense quantities of data, both complex and heterogeneous, and the corresponding evolution of statistical techniques for their analysis and classification. The breakthrough we mentioned may also be due to supercomputers, incredibly powerful machines able to crunch big data in real time.

Among the countless areas where AI can successfully be applied we can mention artificial vision, text and speech recognition, expert systems, robotics, self-driving cars, automatic public-transport operation, even competitive sports.

Oh yes, football too. Nowadays the top clubs make use of mathematics to optimise their performance. During any match of the Italian Serie A, the Spanish Liga or the English Premier League, special cameras record 20–30 times per second the coordinates of the ball and of the 22 players on the pitch. This totals to over 10 million positional data generated during a match. *Big data* algorithms manage to monitor them all, and highlight an enormous number of indicators and useful evaluations. We are not talking about the statistics on ball possession that fill TV programmes at the end of a match, but of instruments capable of reconstructing every single event, like a shot, a pass, a dribble or ball control, all events whose effectiveness mathematics can analyse. AI algorithms can provide in real time operational indications regarding what the manager and their staff want to monitor during the match. It is like having an additional virtual assistant.

The new technologies are revolutionising the labour market as well. According to some analysts, by 2030 AI will create between 555 and 890 million new jobs across the world, and for the same reason 400–800 million people with have to change jobs.

The mathematical abstraction enabling *machine learning* is the *Artificial Neural Network*, made by several decision centres (artificial neurons) connected by logical/mathematical operations that allow to pass from an input to an output without any knowledge of the underlying process. Learning and decision making are developed from the accumulation and comparison of large quantities of data. The network, in practice, is trained to perform certain tasks, and executes them efficiently but without *thinking*. Therefore no new knowledge is created; one only uses the knowledge that can be extracted from the data.

In the light of this, then, AI is complementary to human intelligence, and it is only the latter that oversees the creative act (at least until now: it is difficult to foresee what the future has in store, given the prodigious advances machine learning has made us familiar with in recent years). In describing the world around us, physical laws express exactly the creation of knowledge. These laws are equations and models that do not emerge ``automatically" from the collection of lots of data, but are born out of human reasoning and do not change with the context. Newton's laws, the Navier-Stokes equations, the second principle of thermodynamics are but a few remarkable instances. Once discovered, they become part of the universal heritage, which is invariant in time and space. Put in another way, the model for the atmospheric circulation is valid whether it is applied to the Mediterranean sea, the Arizona desert or the Siberian tundra. The data change, the equations do not. Similarly, the heart model works, in principle, for any human being: it is the data derived from clinical imaging, for example, that will differentiate the heart of one patient from another.

The validity of AI is based on the analysed data, those used for its training. Its results do not permit (yet) the abstraction of laws and models. With this perspective the two approaches may be considered as being alternative. When we examine them more critically (and with more imagination) though, we catch a glimpse of the many opportunities to make them work in a complementary way as well.

I believe, actually, that this path will lead to great progress in the years to come [1].

Reference

1. A. Quarteroni, Algorithms for a New World, Springer Nature, 2022

Printed in the United States
by Baker & Taylor Publisher Services